The Proactive Patient

"*The Proactive Patient* was superbly written! This book is the IC 'bible' for the newly diagnosed as well as the educated patient advocating for quality of life. There isn't another IC book written by an IC patient that has such comprehensive, patient-friendly information. Educating the patient, sharing valuable information such as: IC and overlapping conditions, chemical sensitivities, helpful IC diet tips, and gentle stretching exercises to achieve total body comfort. A must-read for all who want to achieve a full life in spite of having this chronic condition!"

—**Molly Hanna Glidden**, former leader of the Boston MetroWest Interstitial Cystitis Support Group

"I was diagnosed with Interstitial Cystitis and other painful conditions several decades ago. I thought I knew this illness landscape, but *The Proactive Patient* by Gaye and Andrew Sandler taught me how much more there was to learn. I learned something new on every single page of this informative and essential book. You will find everything here—information about diet, traditional and alternative therapies, self-help, managing sex and menopause, and more—all in language that is straightforward and comprehensible to the non-professional. There is also a helpful and touching chapter written by Ms. Sandler's partner and co-author about his role in their shared journey. After enjoying a good read, you will want to keep this book nearby as a valuable resource you will come back to again and again for aid, information, and support."

—**Joy Selak, Ph.D.**, co-author of *You Don't Look Sick! Living Well with Invisible Chronic Illness*

"This book truly is a user's guide to the often misunderstood condition of Interstitial Cystitis. The complex symptoms and pathophysiology are described here in understandable and very thorough detail. By understanding this basis the patient can then explore the vast treatment options, which include both traditional and alternative therapies. I have been a practicing Urologist for 16 years and this book has widened my understanding of IC. I will be recommending it both to my patients and colleagues."

—Joy Nielsen, M.D.

"What sets Gaye and Andrew Sandler apart from so many other authors who have written about interstitial cystitis is their focus on patient comfort. In *The Proactive Patient: Managing Interstitial Cystitis/Bladder Pain Syndrome and the Related Conditions*, they expand upon her previous book by creating a resource guide that will help patients, young and old, as they learn to manage their IC symptoms, reduce pain, age gracefully, and enjoy intimacy again. Every chapter provides the reader (and their family members) with tips and strategies to ease discomfort, control flares, and better manage their symptoms.

"The discussion of traditional therapies is balanced with alternative and complementary therapies for those patients who lack health insurance and/or prefer a more natural approach to treatment. If you, like many others, have faced hostile or unknowledgeable medical care providers, they provide tips on how to find and work with seasoned and compassionate pelvic pain experts.

"Gaye was the first author to explore the relationship between IC and its many related conditions and expands that discussion dramatically in this new book, providing information and self-help tips for patients struggling with IBS, constipation, pelvic floor dysfunction, pudendal neuralgia, fibromyalgia, TMJ, hypothyroidism, and others.

"I particularly appreciated the chapter 'Reclaiming Comfort in Your Body,' which explores exercise ideas, stretching tips, and yoga poses that can help ease discomfort, lessen muscle tension, and regain strength in a pelvic floor compromised by pain, particularly for patients who continue to work and/or who struggle with sitting.

"In recent years, we've learned that chemical sensitivity and environmental illness can play a significant role in the exacerbation of bladder symptoms and general health. This book explores chemical sensitivity and provides a plethora of ideas to help patients reduce toxic exposure and build a toxic-free home, clearly wisdom gained from their own experience with multiple chemical sensitivity. If you plan on remodeling or building a home in the near future, you'll find their suggestions extremely helpful!

"It is in the discussion of hormones, pregnancy, midlife, and sexuality that Gaye and Andrew's work shines. They review, in-depth, the struggles that women face as they age. If you're not sure if hormone replacement therapy is right for you, they provide an excellent discussion of the pros and cons of various hormone treatments. They explore the challenge of intimacy with practical tips on how to reduce discomfort associated with intercourse. Patients exploring pregnancy will find the information on point, even down to the discussion of pros and cons of various delivery methods.

"It is fitting that the book ends with a chapter written by Andrew, titled 'Living with IC/BPS: A Partner's Perspective,' who, with brutal honesty, shares his experience as spouse to an IC patient. He shows how a healthy relationship and family can not only survive but also thrive by creating a foundation of honesty and communication.

"Gaye and Andrew's desire to help others makes them a treasure of the IC movement. Thank you for, yet again, writing a book that will help patients regain their confidence, rebuild their strength, build their knowledge and, most importantly, ease their suffering."

—**Jill Osborne MA**, President of the IC Network

"*The Proactive Patient* is even more resourceful and informative than the authors' first edition, *Patient to Patient*. This new revised edition should be read by every patient who has already been diagnosed, or believes they have IC/BPS and/or one of the related conditions. It should be mandatory reading for all health-care providers—including doctors!—and students learning about the various symptoms and treatments, and especially how you as the patient can more correctly describe your concerns to health-care providers. Most importantly, the health information here will enable you to live a much more active and fuller life. The best proactive patient is the informed patient."

—**Cindy Sinclair**, President, Pure HOPE,
http://www.pure-hope.org/

"Gaye and Andy Sandler have written a very thorough and informative book on PBS/IC. This book will be a valuable addition to the libraries of IC sufferers. Knowledge is certainly power when it comes to living with this debilitating chronic disease. Thanks to Gaye for sharing personal experiences of her journey with IC."

—**Barb Zarnikow**, ICA Patient and Board Co-Chair,
Interstitial Cystitis Association

The Proactive Patient

Managing Interstitial Cystitis / Bladder Pain Syndrome and the Related Conditions

PELVIC FLOOR DYSFUNCTION,
VULVODYNIA, CHRONIC PROSTATITIS,
IRRITABLE BOWEL SYNDROME, FIBROMYALGIA,
AND MORE....

GAYE GRISSOM SANDLER
&
ANDREW B. SANDLER, Ph.D.

Foreword by Robert J. Echenberg, MD, FACOG

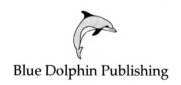

Blue Dolphin Publishing

Published by Blue Dolphin Publishing, Inc.
P.O. Box 8, Nevada City, CA 95959
Orders: 1-800-643-0765
Web: www.bluedolphinpublishing.com

ISBN: 978-1-57733-237-4 paperback
ISBN: 978-1-57733-455-2 e-book

Library of Congress Control Number: 2013952388

Disclaimer: This Work is a result of long-term research and has been reviewed by medical professionals. While every effort has been made to be complete and accurate, new research is ongoing. No part of this book is intended to replace competent medical consultation and treatment. Please consult your personal physician before self-diagnosing.

Cover art:
Painting by Ellen Hermanos Braunstein
Gesture drawing by Katherine Rutledge

Second Edition, January 2015

Printed in the United States of America

5   4   3   2

This book is dedicated to my mother,
June Gripper Grissom,
who taught me through example how to live well
in spite of a chronic illness.

IN MEMORIAM

OF

DR. DANIEL BROOKOFF

a true friend and advocate of the IC/BPS population

CONTENTS

FOREWORD

I was greatly honored to have been contacted some time ago regarding Gaye and Andrew Sandler's request for me to contribute to this work in progress. I received the manuscript recently and marvel now at the enormous research they must have done to write such a definitive work on not just Interstitial Cystitis/Bladder Pain Syndrome (IC/BPS), but on so many of the overlapping conditions that I see on a daily basis in my practice of pain management of the pelvic region.

The science of chronic pain in general and the understanding of the mechanisms of the genetic, neuro-chemical, and the bio-psychosocial underpinnings of myriads of clinical pain disorders has exploded since the 1990s. Correspondingly, and unfortunately, this wealth of new research has been slow in "trickling down" to the variety of medical specialists related to the pelvis.

On the one hand, this book is a wonderfully detailed and sophisticated "self-help" book for all those suffering with IC/BPS and related pain triggering disorders, as well as overlapping disorders, but I honestly believe it should be mandatory reading for all medical students, residents in Urology, Ob/Gyn, Gastroenterology, General and Colo-Rectal Surgery, Orthopedics, Dermatology, etc., as well as in post-graduate fellowship programs such as UroGynecology.

The Sandlers kindly remind the reader that it may be challenging to find health-care practitioners that understand your pain and/or even acknowledge that your "condition" exists. In my own practice I hear those stories on a daily basis. We spend considerable time educating and re-educating our patients about the differences between "acute" and "chronic" pain and how the "dial needs to be turned down" in their central and peripheral and autonomic nervous systems along with diagnosing and treating the "triggering" of that up-regulation, treating those triggers, managing the pain itself, retraining the clenched muscles (specialized pelvic floor physical therapy), and "re-booting" their mid brains not to keep playing the same disturbing and frightening "tapes" of previous injuries and traumas.

It was wonderful to see that this book has not ignored these most important research findings on pain, and even mentions Dr. Daniel Clauw's explanations of chronic pain processing disorders that finally begins to lay out the underlying neuro-pathophysiologies that explain Fibromyalgia and related neuropathic pain disorders. Dr. Clauw has been one of my inspirational thought leaders in my own evolving broader understanding of pain.

Additionally, strong research findings indicate that our bodies, regardless of race, gender, ethnicity, or belief systems, tend to react similarly throughout the world to injury, inflammation, and trauma. Again, this remarkable book did not forget to point out the typical "fight or flight" reactions that are constantly adding to our natural defense mechanisms. We are certainly programmed to automatically and physiologically protect ourselves and our loved ones, even if it might add to our pain and further damage us. Those of us who are parents know that if we were involved in a car accident, and somehow climbed out with a severely fractured leg, but our child is trapped in the car, we would not feel the pain of that injury until we saved our child. The same is obviously true if we injure ourselves falling off a curb, but if a bus is about to hit us, we are still able to run from the danger and the pain comes later. Automatically, and in microseconds, our nervous system tends to make those decisions for us.

In chronic pain, I describe to all of our patients that our tolerance builds gradually in order for us to function with varying degrees of background pain, until that "dial" finally exceeds our tolerance and we go "over the edge" and feel that suddenly we no longer can tolerate even small amounts of discomfort. Young athletes experience what I call "good pain" as they play more and more competitively and commonly learn how to "play through the pain." Unfortunately, many of these young women and men suffer later as they continue to "do life through the pain," and even have "sex through the pain."

Long after previous injuries and traumas have healed, our "muscle memory and nervous system memory" continues to chemically and physiologically "remember" those injuries and traumas. What then can become the "perfect storm" may begin to insidiously bring out more and more of those "memories" especially if common functional, irritating, and often inflammatory disorders are also present. Thus, in the pelvic region we are talking about IC/BPS, IBS, pelvic endometriosis, Vulvodynia, Pudendal Neuralgia, Vulvar Vestibulodynia, and Pelvic Floor Dysfunction, all of which are so much more common than we had ever thought. All of these disorders, along with multiple auto-immune inflammatory disorders (also not uncommon) are the reason so many young women flood to their gynecologists and primary care physicians—and are so commonly misdiagnosed with chronic vaginitis (most commonly "yeast" infections), recurrent ovarian "cysts," and/or "UTIs" in young women and "chronic prostatitis" in young men.

Truly, "everything is connected" when it comes to what is now beginning to be labeled "Chronic Abdominal Pelvic Pain Syndrome" (CAPPS). (I would add to that: "Genital Pain Syndromes" as well.) Simply put, in order to best diagnose and treat these tens of millions of young women and men (in the USA alone), it requires an overview of the whole person and is best done in a setting that is multi-disciplinary, multi-organ system, and involves multi-modal therapies.

Ever since I became interested in pursuing the management of chronic pelvic pain disorders over a decade ago (following over thirty years in Ob/Gyn), I became aware very early on that the bladder pain syndromes were somehow at the "core of the core" related to almost all of these abdominal, pelvic, and genital pain diagnoses. I first concentrated on figuring out how best to diagnose and treat IC/BPS. Dr. Fred Howard from the University of Rochester, a founding member of the International Pelvic Pain Society, wrote an article in one of our journals in 2011, in which he pointed out to all gynecologists that 80 to 85 percent of women with chronic pelvic pain have IC/BPS instead of, or in addition to, a gynecologic reason for their pain. I have had that same experience over the past twelve years. I estimate that I have diagnosed and treated more than 800 women for IC/BPS (and now men as well), for at least a significant portion of the "triggering" of their pelvic regional pain issues.

Another one of my inspirational mentors over the years who helped significantly advance the pain management aspects of IC/BPS has been Dr. Dan Brookoff. He is fondly remembered in this book, and I remember the first time I heard him speak at a pain conference. Dr. Brookoff was a medical oncologist and pain management expert for cancer patients for some time. He recalled in his talk how he became interested in IC/BPS when a female audience member approached him following a talk on cancer pain and asked him to care for her IC/BPS pain. He declined saying he was not a urologist and knew very little about IC/BPS. She persisted in asking for his help and finally told him "she wished she had cancer" so that he would treat her in the same way he had described treating his cancer patients.

I began regularly corresponding with Dr. Brookoff who was always eager to share his knowledge with anyone who cared to hear. He even sent me an unpublished manuscript of a new paper he had written on chronic pain processing in bladder related pain. When I asked him to write the Foreword for my own book, *Secret Suffering: How Women's Sexual and Pelvic Pain Affects Their Relationships*, he immediately agreed and did so. I know the Sandlers join me in remembering such a kind and generous man. We were all deeply saddened by his untimely death just a few years ago.

In closing, I feel that this book, *The Proactive Patient*, should be read by all patients and their caregivers who wish to know almost all there is to know about IC/BPS—including all the extremely helpful personal hints, guidelines, and references that fill so many of its pages. In addition it covers diet, nutrition, manual therapies, overlapping illnesses, chemical sensitivities, sexual and life cycle variables (and more), in a comprehensive manner—certainly not typical of the various previous publications on IC/BPS.

It will definitely be on the reading list for all of my patients. History has often shown that advancements in women's health issues commonly arise from women's own increasing knowledge of their bodies. Providers eventually respond to the demands of their most informed patients. Sadly, as far as these issues are concerned, even now in the twenty-first century, patients still need to become as informed and "proactive" as possible. My hope is that this book will allow each of its readers to explore many different solutions to earlier and more effective care.

Robert J. Echenberg, MD, FACOG
www.instituteforwomeninpain.org

ACKNOWLEDGMENTS

We would like to thank the late Dr. Daniel Brookoff for sharing his research, Dr. Robert Echenberg for his very generous foreword, Dr. Susan McSherry for her expertise, Dr. Randy Birken for his contribution, Dr. Joy Nielsen for her kind testimonial, Dr. Sylvi Beaumont and Dr. Wen Xuan for their contribution, and the following people who also kindly contributed to our book: Jenny Lelwica Buttaccio, Bev Laumann, Ellen Hermanos Braunstein, Katherine Rutledge, Jan North, Rachel Fazio, Jill Osborne, Merrilee Kullman, Barb Zarnikow, Paul Clemens, Mark Shapiro, Diane Wilde, Molly Hanna Glidden, Marilee Nelson, Joy Selak, Cindy Sinclair, and Valerie Barntsen. We are, as well, grateful to Barb Zarnikow's IC/BPS support group, including Catherine Horine, for sharing their experiences and knowledge. We can't forget the love and support of our friends Jo McLean, Melissa O'Brien, and Fenton Rutledge (A.K.A. "Katherine's answering service"), who helped us so much when Gaye's mother was ill toward the end of her life. We truly appreciate all of our friends and family: the Sandler clan, Margaret Einhorn, Frank Khim, Annie Breaux, Debra Brown Grossman, Sally Richards, Margaret Winebrenner, and Becky Wilson for their untiring support and patience, having to repeatedly hear Gaye say (with a sigh), "We have got to finish this book!" Hope we haven't left anyone out.

Chapter One

INTERSTITIAL CYSTITIS/ BLADDER PAIN SYNDROME (IC/BPS)

Interstitial Cystitis/Bladder Pain Syndrome (**IC/BPS**) is a chronic, painful inflammatory condition that affects the bladder wall. Although the symptoms of IC/BPS can mimic an acute urinary tract infection (UTI), the symptoms are not caused by bacteria in the urinary tract. Instead, the symptoms of IC/BPS are believed to be due to abnormalities of the bladder lining (also called the epithelium). Thinning of the lining and changes in the mucous coating of the lining (also called the glycosaminoglycan or GAG layer), that protects the epithelial cells, allow irritants and toxins to permeate and/or cause inflammation of the bladder wall and the exposed nerves. With permeability of the lining (a leaky bladder), deeper cells are also exposed to strong salts and toxic substances. As a result, pain spreads to the surrounding nerves, including the spinal cord, causing a type of neuropathy.

Common Symptoms of IC/BPS

- Pressure in the bladder
- Urgency and urinary frequency up to 80 times a day, including nocturia (frequency during the night)
- Hesitancy when beginning to void
- Decreased and slow urine flow
- Incomplete voiding

- Pain and burning during and/or after voiding
- Sense of relief during and/or after voiding
- Pain in the bladder, in the urethra, and in and around the pelvic area and the supporting muscles of the pelvic floor. In women, IC/BPS pain may occur in the vagina, rectum, and perineum (the area between the anus and vagina). Men may feel IC/BPS pain in the penis, rectum, scrotum, and perineum (the area between the anus and scrotum). (Pain may radiate into the joints and muscles of the low back and sacral area, hips and legs, and affect other areas of the body.)
- IC/BPS symptoms may be misdiagnosed as urethritis in women.
- IC/BPS symptoms may be misdiagnosed as chronic non-bacterial prostatitis (CP/CPPS) in men.

> *Patients may be misdiagnosed if their only symptom is pressure. (Pressure and chronic awareness of the bladder is also considered pain.)*

Over time, without treatment, the IC/BPS bladder may become scarred and stiff, which can limit the capacity to hold urine and empty the bladder completely. But, no matter the size of a patient's bladder (patients can also have enlarged bladders) it is typical for patients to feel the urge to urinate even when their bladders are not full. On occasion, the IC/BPS patient may only experience pain and not frequency. Also unique are the patients who only experience frequency and not pain. Researchers are studying the symptoms and subsets of patients to better understand IC/BPS and how to treat it.

> *IC/BPS does not always progress over time but it may become more difficult to treat as time passes.*

Some patients have a rapid onset of symptoms while others may have mild symptoms, (sometimes called "irritable bladder") for a long period of time. These patients' experience of urgency and incomplete urination may be misdiagnosed until symptoms become chronic. This may happen because IC/BPS symptoms vary patient to patient and can be mild, moderate, or severe. However, the severe bladder pain of IC/BPS inflicts a type of pain only seen in few other medical conditions. IC/BPS pain has been compared to an abscessed tooth, a migraine, ground glass, paper cuts, a lit match, a twisting knife, and acid in the bladder. The pain of IC/BPS has also been likened to reflex sympathetic dystrophy disorder (RSD), a condition that causes chronic regional nerve pain to become a disease in itself.

Several years ago the McGill Pain Inventory, which is a standard medical tool, found the pain of interstitial cystitis to be more severe than the pain of advanced (bladder) cancer. Whatever the symptoms, the pain of IC/BPS can have debilitating effects. Urologists consider IC/BPS and chronic prostatitis/chronic pelvic pain syndrome (CP/CPPS), which produces similar symptoms, the two most disabling disorders they see, not to mention two of the most expensive urological conditions to treat.

Suggested Theories for the Cause of IC/BPS

No one knows what causes IC/BPS. But researchers recognize IC/BPS as a "complex visceral syndrome" which may have a variety of causes. (Visceral refers to the organs—the bladder in the case of IC/BPS.) Several theories for the cause of inflammation and destruction of the bladder wall have been suggested:

- Increased urethral permeability—a defect in the bladder lining (glycosaminoglycan or mucous GAG layer) which allows toxins in the urine to come into contact with the bladder wall causing inflammation of the tissue and exposed nerves (Often the presence of even a small amount of urine causes the bladder to contract.)
- Pathogenic role of mast cells in the bladder (Activation of mast cells plays a part in allergic reactions.)
- Neuroimmune abnormalities (Malfunction of the immune system.)
- Neurological malfunction in either the peripheral or central nervous system which results in inflammation and smooth

muscle dysfunction (The bladder and urethra are in part smooth muscle.)

- Neurological disease process in the nerve roots of the spinal cord
- Toxins remaining in the system after an illness
- Toxic factors in the urine that trigger a low-level autoimmune response
- Hormonal imbalance (Female patients experience flares around cycle changes, perimenopause, and menopause.)
- Pelvic floor dysfunction (PFD)
- Fibromyalgia (FMS) of the bladder
- Irritated nerve endings from previous bacterial infections (Research has shown that IC/BPS may occur after a bladder infection.)
- Nonsteroidal anti-inflammatory drugs (NSAIDs), ibuprofen, and aspirin
- An expression of another disease
- An expression of Lyme disease
- Abnormalities in the neuroendocrine system
- Vulnerability to certain unknown environmental substances

Population Affected by IC/BPS

According to statistics, there are four to 12 million people with IC/BPS in the U.S. Women, men, and children can develop IC/BPS but, so far, 90 percent of all diagnosed patients are female. The usual onset of IC/BPS is thought to occur between 30 to 50 years of age, which makes the average age of the IC/BPS patient 40. Today we know that men, women, and children of all ages, races, cultures, and socioeconomic status can be affected by this condition.

Women in general have more chronic illness. This is probably due to monthly hormones, but some researchers speculate that women have "more developed" limbic systems (the part of the brain that governs emotions) which make women more sensitive. This may be true but does not mean that women's chronic illnesses are psychosomatic.

Understanding the Inflammatory Processes of IC/BPS

Over the years, various treatments have been used to treat the different symptoms of IC/BPS. It's helpful to learn about the inflammatory process of IC/BPS in order to understand how medications and treatments work.

Patients with IC/BPS, and other urogenital pain syndromes often have an increase of nerve density in their bladder walls, specifically sympathetic nerves (which are responsible for a "fight or flight" reaction) and fibers containing substance P. Substance P aids the transmission of pain signals throughout the body and is responsible for the amount of pain one feels. Along with the increase in nerve density, patients may also experience an increase of mast cells in their bladder walls. When mast cell degranulation occurs, as it does in IC/BPS, mast cells release their contents of histamine, leukotrienes, tryptase, as well as other noxious chemicals that are involved in allergic reactions and responsible for vasodilatation, irritation, and inflammation in the surrounding tissues. Degranulation also over-stimulates peptide-secreting sensory nerve fibers and causes the release of nerve growth factor (NGF) and substance P. Substance P in turn furthers the neurogenic (nerve generated) inflammation by re-activating the mast cells and the vicious cycle continues.

Acid-sensing channels (ACIS), found in the IC/BPS bladder, cause excitation, inflammation, and pain in both the peripheral nerves and the central nervous system. They may also be responsible for sensitivity to certain foods. ACIS are typically found in neurological disorders caused by an injury.

Inflammation, allergic and immune reactions, and excitation all play a part in the IC/BPS disease process and cause patients to become hypersensitive to the presence of urine. This hypersensitivity is responsible for the symptoms of IC/BPS.

Nerve growth factor (NGF) and C-reactive protein (CRP) are found in high concentrations in the urine of patients with IC/BPS and chronic prostatitis/chronic prostatitis pain syndrome (CP/CPPS). NGF may become a marker for diagnosis at some point. Similar concentrations of NGF are seen in patients with ulcerative colitis, Crohn's disease, and other inflammatory states. Patients with overactive bladder (OB) have very high levels of NGF but their levels of CRP are lower than the levels found in IC/BPS patients. High levels of substance P are usually found in patients with other chronic pain conditions, including fibromyalgia.

Various Treatments Have Been Used for IC/BPS

According to Jordan Dimitrakov, M.D., Ph.D., and principal investigator of the Genetic Study on IC/BPS, at least 180 different types of therapy have been used for IC/BPS. These therapies include:

- Dietary restrictions—avoiding foods that taste acidic or spicy, foods containing histamines, certain amino acids or amines, flavor enhancers, artificial sweeteners, and preservatives.
- Oral medications to create a protective lining on the bladder wall
- Catheterization of the bladder (with the most comfortable sized catheter) to instill medications that soothe inflammation and repair the bladder lining or act as a temporary replacement for the bladder lining
- Small doses of certain tricyclic antidepressants to block pain and aid sleep
- Antihistamines and combination allergy and asthma medications to suppress mast cell activity
- Pelvic floor therapy to relax hyper-toned muscles
- Electrical stimulation to address nerve inflammation
- Smooth muscle relaxants to calm spasms
- Analgesics to stop burning
- Drugs that block cytokines to prevent inflammation
- Leukotriene inhibitors to reduce allergy and frequency
- Adrenergic blockers to reduce allergy and frequency
- Anti-inflammatory medications to reduce inflammation
- Anticholinergics to decrease urinary frequency

- Medications that combines anticholinergics, antiseptics, antispasmodics, and urinary tract painkillers
- Anti-anxiety medications to calm the pain and aid sleep
- Anti-seizure medications to reduce over-stimulated nerve endings
- Alpha blockers to block pain and relax smooth muscle
- Nerve blocks to prevent painful nerve impulses
- Cox-2 inhibitors to block inflammation
- Toxin injections to paralyze bladder and pelvic floor muscles
- Narcotic antagonists to block mast cell degranulation
- Estrogen-replacement therapy to thicken the bladder lining
- Bladder training to increase the intervals between urination
- Dietary neutralizers and alkalizing agents, and supplements developed specifically for IC/BPS
- Alternative treatments used alone or in conjunction with medical treatments
- Surgery—which is usually considered a last resort

Hyperbaric oxygen, vibration therapy, and hypnosis have proven beneficial to some patients with IC/BPS, fibromyalgia (FMS) and other conditions.

The Cause of IC/BPS Flare-Ups

Because each IC/BPS patient is unique, what bothers one patient does not consistently bother another. But, there are known common irritants. IC/BPS flare-ups are most frequently associated with:

- Diet
- Sexual intercourse
- Menstrual cycle, perimenopause, and menopause
- Allergies and sensitivities to medications and chemicals
- Certain vitamins and supplements
- Seasonal changes, extreme weather conditions, and barometric pressure changes

- Stress, including physical stress like working long hours, standing in lines, lifting and carrying packages, and sitting for long periods
- The wrong type of exercise
- Travel, including riding in a car

Genetic Links/Predisposition

There is a known inherited susceptibility occurring in some families. IC/BPS is found in first-degree relatives, as well as identical twins and multiple generations. Research is ongoing to determine a recessive gene or genes in patients. Other conditions related to IC/BPS may also help researchers to find the genetic link and hopefully the cause of IC/BPS.

> *IC/BPS patients often have overlapping conditions such as irritable bowel syndrome (IBS) or fibromyalgia (FMS), and/or have a family member with an autoimmune condition, such as ulcerative colitis.*

Is IC/BPS Contagious?

No. There is no evidence that IC/BPS is contagious.

IC/BPS Has Been Known to Medicine for a Long Time

The history of IC/BPS is very interesting and very confusing, because this condition has been recognized under several names. IC/BPS was first described by traditional medicine in 1836 as *tic doloureux* of the bladder. The name *tic doloureux* was changed to *interstitial cystitis* in 1887. In 1907, *interstitial cystitis* changed to *cystitis parenchymatosa*. And, when a physician named Guy Hunner discovered ulcers on the bladder wall of a patient in 1915, he changed the name of the condition to *Hunner's ulcer*. Five short years later the name Hunner's ulcer was changed to *panmural ulcerative cystitis*.

Hunner's ulcer is now defined as patches and is still recognized as a condition that affects 5 to 10 percent of all IC/BPS patients.

No matter how many doctors and names have defined IC/BPS, the male oriented field of urology largely continued to consider the condition as a rare disorder of post-menopausal women, as well as a malady caused by hysteria. Hysteria was at that time a diagnosis often used for unexplained symptoms and an array of misunderstood illnesses, predominately affecting women and thought to be caused by repressed emotions. The symptoms of IC/BPS were attributed to emotional problems when urine tests came back negative for infection and there were no signs of Hunner's ulcer. Well beyond the 1950s, repressed emotions were blamed for IC/BPS symptoms and patients underwent many unnecessary surgeries.

Awareness came slowly. In 1958, researchers discovered an increase of mast cells within the bladder walls of IC/BPS patients. They also recognized that Hunner's ulcer was rare in patients and therefore not needed for a diagnosis of IC/BPS. By the mid-1980s workshops, which were held by the National Institute for Diabetes, Digestive, and Kidney Diseases (NIDDK), produced the first guidelines for selecting people for studies of the treatment for what was called *interstitial cystitis.* And, the first diagnostic guidelines were established thanks to prominent urologists.

Still, the trickle down effect from the theory of hysteria lingers in both traditional and alternative medicine. Even though things have vastly improved for IC/BPS patients, it is still not unusual for patients to visit doctor after doctor before finding a correct diagnosis and/or effective treatment.

IC/BPS Research

Research findings and education for both physicians and patients have been available since 1987 thanks in large part to the efforts of non-profit organizations such as the Interstitial Cystitis Association (ICA). The ICA's ongoing advocacy efforts continue to increase research funding by Congress and the National Institutes of Health (NIH).

Experts across the world continue to look for the common cause of IC/BPS. So far, research has shown IC/BPS to be a "symptom complex" with a variety of causes. But the fact that symptoms express differently in patients makes research, diagnosis, and treatment challenging. For example, symptoms may be bladder specific (organ specific) in some patients and centralized (whole-body, systemic) in others. Simply, some patients only experience pain in their bladders and others have widespread symptoms in their whole bodies. Just as some patients show glomerations on their bladder wall (pinpoint bleeding), and others do not.

The fact that all patients are so different has encouraged the phenotyping (classifying) of patients with IC/BPS and chronic prostatitis/chronic pelvic pain syndrome (CP/CPPS), with the hope of finding the appropriate treatments for individual patients, as well as the risk factors for these conditions. Because so many patients have additional urogenital disorders, which respond to the same treatments used for IC/BPS, researchers are now considering these disorders as manifestations of the same disease. The nerves that serve the pelvic organs originate from the same roots in the spinal cord. Simply, pain can transfer from one organ to another and cause an overall pelvic pain pattern when these nerve roots become inflamed. The chronic pelvic pain disorders most associated with IC/BPS are:

- overactive bladder
- pelvic floor dysfunction
- urethral syndrome
- chronic prostatitis (non-bacterial prostatitis)
- vulvodynia
- vulvodynia vestibulitis
- endometriosis
- pudendal (nerve) neuralgia
- irritable bowel syndrome

Patients with overactive bladder (OB), unlike IC/BPS patients, do not experience pressure, and/or pain, with their urgency. Instead, they experience a lack of control.

Also under investigation is the link between IC/BPS and the other medical conditions that overlap in the majority of the IC/BPS population. Researchers hope that these links may point to an immune system disorder. The overlapping conditions being studied are:

- allergies/chemical sensitivity
- fibromyalgia
- chronic fatigue syndrome
- tempomandibular joint disorder
- Sjorgren's syndrome
- Migraine headaches

One of the most important discoveries about IC/BPS occurred over a decade ago when Susan Keay, M.D., Ph.D., Division of Infectious Diseases, University of Maryland School of Medicine, found a revealing, unique protein called antiproliferative factor (APF) in the urine of patients. This peptide appears to be responsible for the thinning of the bladder's protective GAG layer because it inhibits the proliferation (turnover and growth) of new healthy bladder cells and prevents the cells of the lining from sticking together, which is necessary to seal the bladder lining.

Two other factors were found with APF: the heparin-binding epidermal growth factor (HB-EGF) and the epidermal growth factor (EGF), both of which are needed for wound healing. These factors not only appear to be related to APF, they have been found to be decreased in the urine specimens of IC/BPS patients. Today a new bladder instillation of HB-EGF, made from cell cultures, is being tested in patients. It seems the instillation helps the abnormal bladder lining cells change their response to APF and regain their normal function. More clinical trials will be needed but this new treatment could possibly put IC/BPS into remission.

In 2002, the International Continence Society (ICS) established a new term for IC. The Society chose the term "painful bladder syndrome" (PBS) to replace "interstitial cystitis." In the United

States, the term was changed to "interstitial cystitis/painful bladder syndrome" (IC/PBS). But in order to expand the study of overlapping pelvic syndromes associated with IC, the NIH decided to use the umbrella name "urologic chronic pelvic pain syndrome" (UCPPS). To further complicate matters IC is often now referred to in the U.S. as "bladder pain syndrome" (BPS) and/or "chronic abdominal pelvic pain syndrome" which connects everything. See Resources at the end of this chapter to stay current on studies and research information.

Diagnostic Tools

It has taken many years to establish clinical diagnostic guidelines for IC/BPS. The gold standard diagnostic tool for patients has been cystoscopy with hydrodistention, which has also been considered the initial treatment for IC/BPS. During a cystoscopy with hydrodistention, the doctor fills the bladder to its capacity with sterile water and then uses a thin, flexible tube with a light on the end to detect if the patient has glomerulations (tiny strawberry-like hemorrhages) in the bladder wall, as well as inflammation, and/or a thickened, stiff bladder wall. If the doctor detects Hunner's ulcers, the open sores/lesions or patches of well defined inflammation found in the bladder lining, the doctor can vaporize them with a laser wand, electrocautery, or a triamcinolone (a steroid) injection. Doctors typically take a bladder biopsy to rule out cancer.

The cystoscopy must be performed under general anesthesia, otherwise the procedure would be too painful for the IC/BPS patient. (Patients who cannot tolerate general anesthesia may be able to have an epidural instead.) About one third of IC/BPS patients find temporary relief after hydrodistention because sensory nerve fibers are damaged and the bladder is enlarged during the procedure. However, patients usually require strong pain medication for the post-procedure pain. When the doctor cannot find signs of IC/BPS, such as Hunner's ulcers or glomerulations, the condition is diagnosed by the process of exclusion, patient, and family history.

A newer, flexible cystoscope with narrow band imaging may be used to reveal Hunner's ulcers and other dense areas of capillary blood vessels without hydodistention. Although this procedure requires no general anesthesia, some IC/BPS patients may still find it very uncomfortable, if not painful.

New guidelines from the American Urology Association (AUA) suggest a less invasive diagnostic procedure for many patients. The AUA has divided patients into two groups: "uncomplicated" and "complicated." Patients who show "uncomplicated presentations" no longer need to undergo cystoscopy and urodynamics. Instead, urologists or urogynecologists will depend on their clinical judgment to diagnose IC/BPS patients who present the typical discomfort, pressure, or pain in her/his bladder, as well as the symptoms of urgency, frequency, or nocturia. Probably, more than ever, it is essential for IC/BPS patients seeking diagnoses to find urologists or urogynecologists who are familiar with IC/BPS and have worked closely with IC/BPS patients. Not all urologists believe in IC/BPS or want to treat patients with this condition, because treatment is so challenging. (Many urogynecologists are taking over the care of female IC/BPS patients.) Hopefully, these new guidelines will inform and inspire more urologists and urogynecologists, as well as other practitioners, to take an interest in IC/BPS.

Urologists or urogynecologists who are treating patients with "complicated" cases of IC/BPS are still encouraged to perform urodynamics, including cystoscopy with hydrodistention. During urodynamic testing a patient's sensation of bladder fullness is measured along with a reading of urethral pressure to detect pelvic floor hypertonus (overly tight pelvic floor muscles). The doctor will also measure electrical activity of the sphincter and flows of voiding. Urodynamic testing can help a doctor find and treat the cause of a patient's chronic pelvic pain (or incontinence), as well as find and/or rule out other syndromes that occur in the genitourinary system: the pelvis, the colon, and lower spine. (Urodynamics are not specifically used for the diagnosis of IC/BPS.)

Patients who experience any of the following symptoms are considered "complicated."

- Incontinence
- Overactive bladder symptoms
- Blood or pus in the urine (doctors must rule out cancer or look for Hunner's ulcer when blood is found)
- Gynecological or gastrointestinal symptoms

> *IC/BPS does not lead to incontinence, but if a patient does become incontinent it will likely be urgency incontinence and not stress incontinence, which occurs with actions like sneezing or lifting.*

Since men with IC/BPS are often mistakenly diagnosed with chronic prostatitis/chronic pelvic pain syndrome (CP/CPPS), the AUA encourages urologists to look for IC/BPS in men. Although these two conditions are treated differently, urologists should be aware that they can co-exist.

All urologists, urogynecologists, and patients are advised to avoid the potassium sensitivity test because it triggers unnecessary pain and is not always reliable. Until recently, some doctors used this test for both IC/BPS and CP/CPPS to determine if there is a breakdown of the GAG layer that lines the patient's bladder wall. When the GAG layer is permeable (leaky), substances in the urine penetrate the bladder wall, causing irritation. (Not all IC/BPS patients have permeable, leaky bladder linings.) A knowledgeable urologist can usually tell if a patient has a leaky GAG layer by asking which foods and drinks trigger symptoms. For instance, wine is a known irritant. If a patient experiences pain, urgency, and/or frequency after sipping wine, the patient's bladder lining is probably permeable and responsible for the symptoms of IC/BPS.

Another test used to determine if a patient has IC/BPS involves the instillation of the anesthetic lidocaine. If the patient's symptoms decrease after instilling a numbing agent directly into the bladder via catheter, IC/BPS is thought to be the problem. (On occasion, a patient may be sensitive to lidocaine.)

Researchers continue to look for markers in the blood and urine that will make diagnosis easier for both doctors and patients. Some of these markers may reveal the severity of a patent's IC/BPS and lead researchers to new more effective treatments.

New Treatment Guidelines for IC/BPS

The AUA guidelines encourage urologists to begin with more conservative treatments and then move up if needed. This does not imply that a patient with severe symptoms should wait for the most effective treatment. Instead, the initial level of treatment must depend on the severity of the symptoms, as well as a doctor's judgment, and rightfully, a patient's preference. The new guidelines also suggest that urologists practice multimodal therapy (using multiple treatments simultaneously). Treatment options are broken into five lines:

Line One of Treatments:

Self-help, which involves learning as much as possible about IC/BPS, following the special diet, completely avoiding Kegel exercises, modifying lifestyle to reduce stress, and treating overlapping conditions that aggravate the bladder, is considered the first line of treatment. *Refer to Chapter Two and Chapter Seven for more information on diet and self-help.*

Line Two of Treatments:

Doctors are advised to begin their "uncomplicated patients" with conservative treatment, which may include appropriate physical therapy *(see Chapter Four)*, and the medications: Tagamet (cimetidine), Elavil (amitriptyline), Atarax or Vistaril (hydroxyzine), Elmiron (pentosan polysulfate), DMSO (dimethyl sulfoxide), lidocaine, and heparin.

- **Tagamet (cimetidine)** is an over-the-counter oral antihistamine (a histamine 2 blocker), as well as a stomach acid-blocker. H2 blockers appear to calm the bladder as well as the gut and, according to some doctors, may work better for symptoms than H1 blockers. Tagamet tablets and liquid

Tagamet contain inactive ingredients that may trigger bladder symptoms in some patients.

- **Elavil (amitriptyline)** is an older oral tricyclic antidepressant (TCA) often prescribed in low doses for pain syndromes (low dose antidepressants prescribed to reduce pain do not affect one's mood or depression). Many patients have benefited from amitriptyline's analgesic and antihistamine actions, as well as its sedative effects. As a matter of fact, amitriptyline is made of five medications which appear to help with the different symptoms of IC/BPS. This medication is recommended to be taken at bedtime when it helps to combat nocturia; however, a small percentage of patients prefer to take it earlier in the evening for two reasons. The first reason is because amitriptyline can have a temporary stimulating effect before a sedating one, and the second reason being that the drowsy effects can sometimes last through the next morning if taken too late the night before.

  The usual side effects include dry mouth, constipation, dry skin, sun sensitivity, weight gain, sweating, and decreased blood pressure. Amitriptyline is sometimes helpful to patients with the diarrhea type of irritable bowel syndrome (IBS-D), and with migraine headaches and fibromyalgia.

- **Atarax and Vistaril (hydroxyzine)** are tricyclic H1 blocker antihistamines and mild anti-anxiety medications. Hydroxyzine (Atarax or Vistaril) is used to block mast-cell secretion, which stimulates swelling and inflammation in the tissues of the bladder. It works well to decrease pain and frequency because it counteracts allergic reactions and helps to block the neurotransmitter acetylcholine. (Vistaril may have a slightly higher rate of absorption.) Most patients begin with a small dosage of hydroxyzine, 10 mg. at bedtime, then slowly increase the dosage up to 75 mg. over a period of one month. Patients may notice improvement in a few weeks or a few months. Hydroxyzine also helps patients with allergies, migraines, and IBS. Side effects of all antihistamines include dry mouth, drowsiness, and weight gain. A liquid form can be prescribed for individual patients sensitive to the fillers and/or dyes found in capsules and pills. Because of hydroxyzine's sedating effects, it is best taken at night. Patients who are allergic to acacia should avoid Atarax. All patients should avoid antihistamines containing decongestants.

- **Elmiron (pentosan polysulfate)** is the first FDA approved oral treatment developed for IC/BPS. Elmiron is a heparin binding compound that enhances the GAG layer by "filling in the gaps." The bladder lining is made of a protective glucosamine and Elmiron has chemical similarities to chondroitin and glucosamine. Elmiron is also known to have anti-inflammatory properties that decrease oversensitization in the bladder, which results in less frequency and pain. Some scientists suggest that this medication may act as an inhibitor of growth factors and free radicals, and may possibly provide a barrier against bladder infections.

  The chief side effects of Elmiron are diarrhea, nausea (thought to be caused by the capsule), and headache. Stomach upset can usually be avoided by pouring the medication out of the capsule and into water. A small number of patients may also experience hair loss and rash. The recommended dosage is 100 mg. 3 times a day, but the late IC/BPS pain specialist, Daniel Brookoff, M.D., believed it to be more beneficial for patients to take 300 mg. twice a day on an empty stomach instead. Patients are advised to discontinue Elmiron three months before surgery, because Elmiron acts as a heparoid and heparin is a known blood thinner.

  Typically, patients take Elmiron in conjunction with other medications because results can take up to 8-12 weeks (the full effect may take up to six months). Successful results may depend on how long a patient has had IC/BPS. Newer IC/BPS patients appear to have more success with Elmiron than those with a long history of IC/BPS. Elmiron can also be instilled into the bladder and/or made into a cocktail with sodium bicarbonate and a steroid, but because it causes burning and has proven unhelpful to patients, very few doctors use Elmiron instillations. (Occasionally, a patient may experience a worsening of symptoms with sodium bicarbonate.)

- **DMSO (dimethyl sulfoxide) (RIMSO-50)** has been used as a bladder instillation for many years. Bladder instillations have been considered the most direct method to treat bladder inflammation. DMSO via catheter is a standard treatment for IC/BPS, although there are some urologists who feel it is too invasive for patients. Nevertheless, many patients experience relief with this anti-inflammatory. The properties of DMSO have analgesic and antihistamine effects and encourage muscle relaxation, as well. DMSO is helpful to both the ulcerous (Hunner's ulcer) and non-ulcerous forms of IC/BPS and has a 50 to 70 percent improvement rate in ulcerous IC/BPS.

  DMSO has been on the fringe of medically accepted treatments for arthritis for years and was the first drug approved for the treatment of IC/BPS. DMSO instillations are absorbed into the bloodstream through the mucous membrane lining of the bladder. Patients experience a garlic-like taste and breath, and sometimes flu-like symptoms, and/or a worsening of symptoms a day or two after treatment. Uncomfortable symptoms are thought to be caused by temporary histamine release from mast cells, the release of substance P (an inflammatory mediator), and chemical burn. If a patient finds DMSO too irritating, the DMSO can be cut in half with sterile water and still used in a cocktail if needed. (Adding a steroid may also reduce the burning sensation and offer more relief.) Patients usually notice improvement after their third instillation. However, there are patients who don't experience improvement until a full month after a cycle of treatments.

  Follow-up treatments for recurring symptoms depend on individual needs. If a patient chooses to self-catheterize her or his medications, urine should be tested before instillation to rule out a urinary tract infection (UTI). Most patients prefer pediatric catheters because larger adult catheters create additional pain. On the other hand, there are patients who prefer the adult catheter because it offers less dwell time (the length of time that the catheter is in place).

DMSO is sometimes used to carry other medications and is often mixed with other medications to make a bladder cocktail. Solutions such as hydrocortisone (a steroid), lidocaine (a short-lived anesthetic), marcaine (a long-lasting anesthetic), and/or heparin (which mimics the bladder's mucous lining) can be added to the DMSO to make a cocktail or used alone to soothe inflammation. Sodium bicarbonate and/or an antibiotic may also be added to the DMSO, but not all patients respond well to sodium bicarbonate or antibiotics. When a patient has a bad reaction to a cocktail, the doctor may not know which ingredient has irritated the patient's bladder. In this situation a patient can ask to re-start with just one or two ingredients to detect which, if any, ingredients are irritating.

Patients must only use RIMSO-50 DMSO, and it should not be held more than 15 to 20 minutes per treatment because a longer "dwell time" may damage tissue and/or deliver systemic absorption. To date, there have been no serious side effects reported, but patients were recommended in the past to have periodic ophthalmologic slit-lamp examinations, blood counts, and kidney and liver function tests a few times a year.

> *It has been suggested that steroid instillations eventually thin the bladder lining but many patients have used steroid instillations alone or mixed with DMSO, or another solution, for years and have reported relief.*

- **Lidocaine instillations** are used for their anesthetic effect to calm inflammation, for their ability to increase bladder capacity, urine flow, and the length of time between voids, and possibly their ability to help prevent urinary tract infections (UTIs). Lidocaine and other anesthetics have been used as "rescue instillations" for those patients in a flare-up and also as a series of treatments. Some urologists use alkalinized lidocaine (PSD597), which is lidocaine mixed with sodium bicarbonate. The bicarbonate is meant to improve the lidocaine absorption, as well as decrease severe pain. IC/BPS patients who cannot tolerate, or notice no improvement with sodium bicarbonate or lidocaine, may try bupivacaine (Marcaine). Marcaine is a longer-acting anesthetic that can also be used as a bladder instillation, and like lidocaine, it can be mixed with other medications in cocktails. These bladder instillations can also be used for long-term control of symptoms.

- **Heparin** is a natural substance found in the body. Its purpose is to prevent blood clotting in the veins. Heparin sodium is a medication that mimics the bladder's GAG because it has chemical similarities to chondroitin and glucosamine. Instillations of heparin are given in a series to coat the bladder and calm inflammation. Urologists often use heparin alone or mixed into a bladder cocktail. An instillation named URG101 contains both heparin and alkalinized lidocaine. Doctors have different opinions about mixing heparinoid drugs; some believe that heparin should not be mixed with lidocaine and/or bicarbonate.

> *Female patients should avoid stirrups while holding a bladder instillation. Maintaining the position in stirrups for 15 minutes or more can result in low-back and hip pain. Instead, the exam table should be extended to support bent knees and flat feet if patients choose to lie down during dwell time.*
>
> *Sitting on the end of an exam table also presents a problem. Many gynecological tables have a slight tilt for examination purposes. Sitting on this tilt causes the pelvis to roll into a posterior position (back and under), which can also lead to low-back and hip pain. It's best to sit on a chair or on the side of the table while waiting for the doctor or nurse.*

Line Three of Treatments:

When a doctor suspects a patient has Hunner's ulcer and wants to rule out cancer or other suspected conditions because of blood in the urine, **cystoscopy** under anesthesia with hydrodistention is recommended. *See Diagnostic Tools.*

Line Four of Treatments:

Neuromodulation, which is suggested as the fourth option of treatment, is electrical nerve stimulation via the sacral nerves or the tibia nerve. Sacral neuromodulation stimulates the sacral nerve roots that serve the pelvis and can be used to treat patients with IC/BPS and/or CP/CPPS. (There is some evidence that certain neuromodulation may also help some patients with vulvodynia and IBS.) Stimulation of the third sacral nerve appears to decrease frequency, increase bladder capacity and blood flow to the bladder, increase urinary concentrations of heparin-binding epidermal growth factor-like growth factor, and reduce concentrations of the anti-proliferative factor, which is the urinary marker associated with the symptoms of IC/BPS. The favorable form of neuromodulation for IC/BPS is a device called **InterStim**. This implantable device is typically used to treat urinary urge incontinence and urgency-frequency syndrome. Although InterStim is only approved for the treatment of bladder-control problems, it also helps IC/BPS patients whose predominant symptoms are urgency and frequency. InterStim is not recommended for patients whose main symptom is pain. Nor is it considered a first line treatment for IC/BPS. Only patients who show improvement with the initial test are eligible for this treatment.

The InterStim test involves placing an electrode in the third sacral nerve (S3) area and then connecting it to an external impulse generator. The patient has control to turn it on or off, as well as up or down. If the patient experiences improvement, she or he is eligible for full implantation, which is placed just under the skin in the buttocks. Although rare, there are patients who experience greater relief with "bilateral stimulation," which requires two devices, one in each buttock. Or, some patients benefit from a "single bilateral" device, which works like having the two implants.

The possible side effects of InterStim are abdominal pain, infection, lead migration, and possible sensitivity to the implant. Patients with InterStim implants should avoid activities that put them at risk for a high-impact fall. Such a fall may cause damage to the device or dislocate the lead wire. Fixing these damages requires surgery in order to replace or re-position the wire or device.

> *The InterStim device is sealed with silicone rubber, which may touch tissue when implanted. Medtronic, the maker of Inter-Stim, offers a test to detect a patient's reaction to the InterStim device. If a patient cannot tolerate the device, it can be changed to accommodate the patient.*

The first commercial tibia stimulation, called the Stoller Afferent Nerve Stimulation (SANS), was a form of e-stim approved for urgency and frequency. In recent years, a newer updated device, called the **Urgent PC neuromodulation system**, has been approved for overactive bladder. Like SANS, this new tibial stimulation device can also be used for IC/BPS and is considered to be less invasive than the other forms of neurostimulation.

During the 30-minute treatment, the doctor or physical therapist inserts a small slim needle, similar to an acupuncture needle, near the tibial nerve above the ankle. The needle is then connected to a battery-powered stimulator, which sends impulses to the tibia nerve and on up to the sacral area that controls bladder function.

The standard number of treatments for overactive bladder (OAB) is 12. OAB patients, who have success with the Urgent PC, usually feel results halfway through the treatments. They can return as needed after the initial 12 treatments. IC/BPS patients appear to need more than the standard initial treatments to achieve and/or maintain improvement. Side effects of the Urgent PC include discomfort or bleeding at the needle site. Patients need to use good back support during the treatments, which require patients to sit and rest the treated leg up on a block or chair. If hip or low back pain occurs, a standard-size towel can be folded in half and placed under the buttock opposite the lifted leg. (This is an Aston-Patterning modification technique. Aston-Patterning is a sophisticated form of muscle and movement re-education.)

Line Five of Treatments:

The AUA recommends the immunosuppressant **cyclosporine** and **Botulinum Toxin A** (Botox) as options for the fifth line of treatment. Cyclosporine (Sandimmune) is an immunosuppressant peptide that is produced by an extract of soil fungi. Cyclosporine inhibits lymphocytes (white blood cells that are responsible for immune responses) by suppressing the immune system.

Botulinum Toxin is typically used for overactive bladder that leads to incontinence. It works by paralyzing the detrusor muscle which helps to empty the bladder during urination. In IC/BPS patients, Botox can be injected into the lower bladder (which is mostly responsible for sensations) to stop contractions of the muscle and the release of sensory transmitters that promote abnormal pain sensations.

Before injecting a patient with Botox, the doctor uses an anesthetic block as a test. If the anesthetic injection is helpful, the doctor will repeat the injection with Botox. In patients with PFD, Botox can be injected into trigger points of the major pelvic-floor muscles. Pelvic-floor therapy can enhance relaxation of the muscles after injection. Botox is not considered a standard treatment for IC/BPS patients. A patient must go under anesthesia for this treatment and may need to self-catheterize for a long period of time after treatment.

Line Six of Treatment:

Major surgery to remove the bladder, enlarge the bladder, or create urinary diversion is considered as a last resort for patients with the severe and unremitting pain of advanced IC/BPS. Surgery, however, is reserved for only the most severe cases of IC/BPS, but may be necessary when a patient's pain and frequency become unbearable and the bladder becomes scarred, stiff, and diminished in size, reducing the capacity to hold urine.

After surgery, some IC/BPS patients do feel better, but different types of surgeries offer different results. IC/BPS patients still stand the chance of continued pain if the bladder neck, trigone (the base of the bladder where there is a concentration of nerves), and urethra are left in place. Patients may even experience phantom pain after surgery. Other risks include chronic infections of the bladder and kidney, incontinence, and the need to self-catheterize. Small bowel obstruction or spontaneous rupture can occur with an intestinal pouch.

With **augmentation surgery,** the bladder is made larger by adding a section of the patient's bowel. Only the scarred, ulcerated, and inflamed sections of the patient's bladder are removed, leaving the healthy tissue and the base of the bladder intact. A piece of the patient's bowel can be removed, reshaped, and then attached to the remaining healthy tissue of the bladder. The patient may be able to void normally with the bladder substitution after the incisions are healed. Even in select patients with small and contracted bladders, the symptoms of pain, frequency, and urgency may continue or return after surgery. In some instances, the disease process of IC/BPS may affect the new tissue made from the section of the bowel. Patients may also be at risk for incontinence or the opposite: the inability to void at all. When this is the result of surgery, the patient must use a catheter to empty urine from her or his bladder.

Different methods of urinary diversion can be used to reroute urine after the bladder has been removed. In most cases, the ureters (the tubes that carry urine from the kidneys to the bladder) are attached to a piece of the bowel that connects and opens to the outside of the abdomen. The urine empties through the stoma, the opening in the abdomen, into a bag outside the body. This procedure is called a **urostomy** and helps to eliminate the frequency, but not the pain, of IC/BPS.

Some urologists use an internal pouch, which also requires a stoma, but the urine is stored inside the abdomen in a pouch. The patient must put a catheter into the stoma and empty the internal pouch several times a day. With either type of urostomy, a patient must take very clean and sterile measures to prevent infections in and around the stoma.

Another type of urinary diversion involves making a new bladder from a piece of the patient's bowel. The new piece is attached to the urethra after the bladder has been removed. The patient can then urinate normally through the urethra, but may be at risk for urinary incontinence after this type of diversion.

The AUA Advises Doctors and Patients to Avoid:

- Long-term antibiotics
- Bacillus Calmette-Guerin (BCG) instillations
- High-pressure and long-duration hydrodystention
- Long-term oral steroids
- Urethral dilation
- Urethrotomy

> *The painful and caustic bladder instillations of chlorpactin and silver nitrate are no longer approved for clinical use. Neither is the bladder instillation RTX (resiniferatoxin), which was proposed as a candidate for IC/BPS treatment. Many doctors are also moving away from DMSO and steroid instillations. Other medicines, such as heparin and numbing agents, are now taking their place.*

Pain Management Options Not Mentioned in the AUA Guidelines

The AUA emphasizes the importance of symptom and pain management, and there are other treatments that have helped the occasional patient. For example, Zantac (ranitidine) is also a histamine 2 blocker and an alternative to Tagamet. (Patients should avoid Zantac Effervescent Tablets because they contain the bladder irritant aspartame.) Alternatives for the H1 blockers Atarax and Vistaril are over-the-counter Benadryl (diphenhydramine), which aids sleep, Zrytec (cetirizine), the oral preparation of Gastrocrom (cromolyn sodium), and the nasal spray version of this medication, Nasalcrom, both typically used to relieve asthma and allergies and, sometimes, irritable bowel syndrome (IBS), and the leukotriene inhibitor Singulair (montelukast), which has been found to reduce frequency and pain in some IC/BPS patients.

Patients who find they cannot tolerate amitriptyline may benefit from one of the other tricyclic antidepressants (TCAs), such as Sinequan (doxepin), Pamelor (nortriptyline), and Tofranil (imipramine). (Nortriptyline is available in liquid form.) Newer SSRIs (selective serotonin reuptake inhibitors), SSRNIs (selective serotonin and norepinepherine reuptake inhibitors), and SNRIs (selective norepinepherine reuptake inhibitors) do not seem to reduce symptoms like the tricyclic antidepressants, and some cause symptoms to flare-up.

When patients need immediate relief, anticholinergics, antispasmodics, and bladder analgesics can often calm symptoms. Anticholinergics combined with antispasmodics, such as Ditropan XL (oxybutynin), Urised, a drug combination of an antibacterial, an analgesic and anticholinergic, and Levsin (hyoscyamine), also an antiseptic, can control frequency and urgency, and increase bladder capacity. Drugs that act as bladder analgesics, such as Pyridium (phenazopyridine), Urelle, and over-the-counter Uristat and Azo Standard, are often prescribed for burning. Muscle relaxants, such as Valium (diazepam) and Flexeril (cyclobenzaprine), both benzodiazepenes, can be taken to stop bladder contractions (some patients report an increase in bladder symptoms with Flexeril).

Pyridium is intended for short-term use. Long-term use can destroy red blood cells made by bone marrow.

Valium is known to be effective on both striated and smooth-muscle and therefore acts as a relaxant for the pelvic floor. Strong dosage is usually needed to aid sleep in patients with nocturia (night-time frequency). Valium can also be compounded into vaginal suppositories which may prevent exercise induced pain, as well as pain after intercourse (dyspareunia). Oral Valium can also be inserted intravaginally, but patients should discuss this with their doctor before trying this method. Other vaginal suppositories that can be compounded for patients include the anesthetic lidocaine, the antidepressant amitriptyline, or the anticonvulsant Neurontin (gabapentin). None of these medications are intended for rectal use.

> *A new small lidocaine-releasing device (that is placed in the bladder) is being studied. Patients call it "the pretzel."*

Oral anti-seizure medications are another option to treat IC/BPS. The anticonvulsant Neurontin is mainly used for epileptic seizures, but can calm hyper-excitability of the nerves in people with chronic pain and neurogenic (nerve generated) conditions, such as IC/BPS, CP/CPPS, IBS, and FMS. Neurontin not only calms the over sensitization, but also the spinal nerve damage which generates the neuropathic pain and inflammation in the bladder. It is usually taken three times a day, but some doctors prefer that their patients begin with two daily doses. Either way, patients must start with small doses. The side effects of Neurontin are sleepiness and dizziness, other nervous system effects, and water retention. Patients are advised to stay well hydrated. Although rare, some patients report a worsening of their IC/BPS symptoms after taking anti-seizure medications.

Lyrica (pregabalin) is another anti-seizure medication that can be prescribed for IC/BPS symptoms, but again not all patients can tolerate this medication. Anti-seizure medications are often used in conjunction with other complementary therapies.

Aside from the bladder instillations listed in Line Two of the AUA Guidelines, there a few other options that may help some patients: Cystistat (hyaluronic acid), which requires a long dwell time, Cytotec (misoprostol), a drug that is used to regenerate the cells of the lining of the gastrointestinal tract, and Uracyst (chondroitin sulfate), which is a glycosaminoglycan (GAG).

Newer bladder washes and instillations are getting attention. One such instillation is honey. Honey has been used for centuries as a wound-healer and a component in honey has proven beneficial in soothing IC/BPS symptoms. Soothing and long-lasting liposomes are another example. These types of fat globule can be instilled alone to create a protective barrier from irritating substances and/or used to encapsulate and deliver other medications, such as a cannabinoid drug.

> *Liposomes are nanoparticles, which are presently considered controversial. There are concerns about the effects that nanoparticles may cause if they are absorbed into the bloodstream.*

New drugs that target, block or activate receptors in the bladder are being investigated. Receptors respond to stimulus and send signals, both good and bad, to the central nervous system. They also act to relax and contract the bladder. Various types of receptors are found in the bladder, such as the opioid receptors, estrogen receptors, vanilloid receptors, and cannabinoid receptors. Some researchers are actually looking at the value of marijuana (cannabis) and its active components (cannabinoids) for the treatment of IC/BPS.

Cannabinoids appear to suppress the behavioral response to the pain-related chemicals that are released in the inflammatory process of IC/BPS. Cannabinoids also contain antispasmodic and analgesic properties that affect the central and peripheral nerves, both of which are involved in IC/BPS. As of yet, researchers have not studied cannabinoids in IC/BPS patients, but they have had a lot of positive feedback from patients who have tried medical marijuana. These patients report less urgency and frequency, less pain and better sleep, along with other comforting benefits. Patients who must take opioids may be able to lower the dosage of their medication because marijuana enhances the effects of opioids. Other patients may be able to replace their opioids with marijuana. Still, in order to better understand which cannabinoids may help IC/BPS patients, the different strains of the plant need to be investigated.

Although medical marijuana remains illegal in most states, a cannabis-like medication may be available in the future. A cannabinoid drug is presently being studied in the treatment of chronic prostatitis/chronic pelvic pain syndrome (CP/CPPS) and this new drug is scheduled to be studied in IC/BPS patients next.

Until better pain management is available, the IC/BPS patient, who has exhausted most therapies, must turn to stronger medication to treat bladder pain. Short-acting opioid medications, such as Percodan (oxycodone combined with aspirin), Percocet (oxycodone combined with acetaminophen), Vicodin and Lortab (hydrocodone combined with acetaminophen) for analgesic properties, can help calm bladder pain during an acute flare-up. But not all doctors are comfortable prescribing opioids, so when a pain cycle cannot be stopped, and a patient is in chronic, severe, and debilitating pain day after day, she or he will usually need to see a pain specialist.

Anyone who has taken a course of opiods is familiar with the side effect of chronic constipation. Whether the IC/BPS patient can tolerate this particular drug is questionable, but the inject-able laxative Relistor (methylnaltrexone bromide) helps bowel function in those taking opioid pain medications.

Doctors who specialize in chronic pain management know that patients who suffer with chronic pain do not experience the "high" and craving of a drug addict. Instead, patients experience relief from narcotics. Although the body can develop a natural tolerance to a drug, a patient who is severely disabled by daily pain may find relief with a small, steady, slow release of pain medication through a localized patch, such as a Duragesic (fentanyl) transdermal patch, a morphine pump, or an oral dose of long acting opiods like Demerol (meperidine), methadone, or a belladonna and opium (B&O) rectal suppository, which provides relief for prostate pain and urethral spasm, as well as other painful symptoms.

Rarely, belladonna can over-relax the bladder causing pain and the inability to empty the bladder.

A pain specialist can also help design a plan for fast-acting rescue opioids to treat breakthrough pain when a patient is on a long-acting opioid medication schedule. Or, a specialist can prescribe a compounded topical prescription of non-opiod Ketamine (which should be available as a nasal spray soon). Ketamine is helpful to some patients with severe breakthrough pain; however, people who abuse Ketamine as a recreational drug can actually injure their bladders.

Therapeutic treatments must always be monitored closely because there is often a fine line between pain control that can improve the quality of life, and the side effects of pain medication that can interfere with the quality of life. Each IC/BPS patient presents individual needs and challenges to the doctor.

*Electrical stimulation (e-stim) has been a drug-free option for years for patients with chronic pain. The different forms of e-stim may offer some IC/BPS patients another form of self-help. The **TENS** unit (transcutaneous electrical nerve stimulation) is one of the oldest forms of nerve stimulation. In the case of IC/BPS patients, the unit is placed above the bladder or on the lower back to stimulate hormones that block pain, increase blood flow to the bladder, and strengthen the pelvic muscles. TENS has also been beneficial for patients with Hunner's ulcer. Side effects of the unit include skin irritation from the adhesive. The **EMPIIF3 WAVE** is like the TENS unit, but 50 times stronger. Worn on a belt, it has a specific program for IC/BPS and is designed to promote pelvic floor relaxation, relieve urinary urgency and/or prostatic pain, as well as sex and exercise-induced pain. (Other forms of e-stim have been explored for the treatment of IC/BPS.)*

Natural Supplements Used For IC/BPS

Several companies have made natural supplements to improve bladder health; other companies have discovered that their supplements help patients with IC/BPS and/or CP/CPPS. Refer to the following:

- **CystoProtek**, an oral dietary supplement developed by Theoharis Theoharides, M.D., Ph.D., and his colleague, urologist Grannum R. Sant, M.D., contains the anti-inflammatory properties of chondroitin sulfate, quercetin, and rutin. Quercetin is naturally found in plants and seeds, and contains anti-oxidant and anti-inflammatory properties which block the release of histamines. These properties, along with other beneficial ingredients, help restore the GAG layer of the bladder, calm mast cells, and reduce pain. Some patients find that the capsule irritates their bladders, so they empty the contents from the capsule and mix the contents with juice or food.

- **Cysta-Q** and **Prosta-Q** are over-the-counter dietary supplements formulated to reduce IC/BPS urgency, frequency, and pain. Prosta-Q promotes prostrate health and reduces symptoms of CP/CPPS in men. The main ingredient in these supplements is quercetin, which is blended with bromelain and several herbs and plants.

- **Prelief** (calcium glycerophosphate) is an over-the-counter supplement used to reduce heartburn and acid in the stomach. It also helps to reduce bladder pain, urinary frequency and urgency, and acts as a neutralizer when taken with food. A new study has shown that Prelief has some wound-healing properties. Prelief can be found in grocery and drug stores.

- Desert Harvest makes a supplement designed just for IC/BPS patients. **Desert Harvest Aloe Vera** can be used during a flare-up or as a preventative supplement to reduce urinary frequency, burning, and pain in both IC/BPS and CP/CPPS patients. The main ingredient of this supplement is glycosaminoglycans (GAGs). Depending on the strength, aloe vera offers natural anti-inflammatory, antibiotic, analgesic, and anti-microbial agents. Patients should avoid Desert Harvest Liquid Aloe Vera, as it contains citric acid.

Other over-the-counter supplements that act to enhance the GAG layer of the bladder include CystoRenew, Bladder-Q, and Bladder Ease. Probiotics, specifically engineered to suppress the pain of IC/BPS and recurring urinary tract infections, may be available in the future.

Overlapping Conditions and Symptoms

For years many IC/BPS patients and their doctors have felt that IC/BPS is more than a bladder disease. IC/BPS often appears as a multi-faceted disease that affects the whole person. When this is the case, IC/BPS is considered systemic and not organ-specific (just affecting the bladder), but some experts wonder if IC/BPS is a localized syndrome of a disease that affects the whole body. Perhaps a clue to this question will depend on whether a patient has one of the related conditions before IC/BPS or developed one of the conditions after IC/BPS. Whatever researchers eventually conclude, the connection to the overlapping symptoms and conditions is becoming clearer. The most common related conditions are:

Pelvic Floor Dysfunction (PFD)

The pelvic floor is a muscular hammock-like structure that supports the internal pelvic organs. When a person has pelvic floor dysfunction (PFD), her or his pelvic floor muscles don't contract and relax normally. PFD causes pain and inflammation in patients with IC/BPS and chronic prostatitis (CP/CPPS), as well as other related syndromes. Sometimes PFD is called prostatodynia in men. The spasms from this condition can lead to urinary urgency, constipation, and painful sexual intercourse. Trigger points in the pelvic floor, which may be caused by IC/BPS and CP/CPPS, further the irritation and cause a vicious cycle. Medications, such as low dose Valium, may be taken to relax the pelvic floor. Trigger-point therapy is also helpful, as are relaxation techniques, warm sitz baths, and the right type of exercise. *Refer to Chapters Three and Four.*

> *Female IC/BPS patients should ask their doctors or nurses to use a pediatric speculum for their pelvic exams. Also helpful is to have the doctors or nurses turn the speculum blades sideways.*

Irritable Bowel Syndrome (IBS)

In a large survey of IC/BPS patients 64 percent said they also suffered with irritable bowel syndrome (IBS). This came as no surprise to the researchers who found that there is a cross-talk between the colon and the bladder due to their shared nerve pathway. Now known as "cross-sensitization," foods which irritate the colon can in turn irritate the bladder and vice-versa. This makes a lot of sense to the patients who sometimes can't distinguish which organ is causing pelvic pressure. Other contributing factors that lead to abnormal organ function and irritation are the mast cells that migrate between the colon and bladder, and the problematic trigger points in the pelvic floor and abdomen.

IBS is considered a sensory disorder that mostly affects women; however, many men with CP/CPPS are also affected with the condition. IBS causes bloating, cramping, gas, passage of mucous, and bouts of diarrhea or constipation, as well as upper GI symptoms and bladder symptoms in IC/BPS patients. Suggested causes of IBS in the general public are disturbances in the muscles or nerves in the colon, and/or a hypersensitivity in the brain to bowel sensations. Since more than 90 percent of the body's serotonin (a neurotransmitter that sends messages between nerve cells) is found in the lining of the gut, some experts believe that IBS is caused by an imbalance of serotonin. They think that patients who mostly suffer with diarrhea-prominent IBS have increased serotonin levels in their gut, and patients who suffer with constipation-predominant IBS have decreased amounts of serotonin. However, sometimes IBS can be triggered by an intestinal virus.

IBS can cause referred pain to the low back, hips, and legs, and can worsen with the hormonal swings of the menstrual cycle. Although a tricyclic antidepressant, like amitriptyline or desipramine, can be helpful to patients who suffer with diarrhea (IBS-D), tricyclic antidepressants may worsen symptoms in patients who suffer with constipation (IBS-C). The SSRI medication Lexapro is also known to help patients with IBS-D, but SSRI drugs are not always tolerated by IC/BPS patients. Although there is a prescription medication designed to relieve IBS-D named Lotronex, it is not known if it will trigger bladder symptoms in IC/BPS patients. Today, researchers are studying an amino acid called glutamine, which may help patients with IBS-D. Amitiza (lubiprostone), a drug developed for chronic constipation and bloating, may also help patients with IBS-C, if tolerated. (Some patients do fine with Amitiza.)

A safer approach to treating IBS symptoms for IC/BPS patients includes treating trigger points in the pelvic floor and abdomen, taking a low dose of a probiotic, such as Klaire Labs Pro-Biotic Complex (if tolerated), and modifying one's diet and lifestyle. *Refer to Chapter Two.*

> *Although doctors who treat patients with IBS say that their patients have both bouts of constipation and diarrhea, some researchers believe that around a third of all patients with IBS have IBS-D. Another third have IBS-C and the remaining third suffer with both types of the condition. (It appears that patients with IBS-D are more likely to have increased intestinal permeability, which is called leaky gut.)*

Fibromyalgia (FMS)

FMS affects a large population of IC/BPS patients and appears to be a chronic disease of neurohormonal abnormalities in the brain that affect sensory processing, cause immune system changes, and make patients feel like they have a virus. Like many other chronic pain conditions, including IC/BPS, FMS triggers grey matter changes in patients' brains, referred to as "fibro fog." When the brain and/or spinal cord can't process pain signals properly, the threshold to pain is lowered. This is called central sensitization. Exaggerated perceptions of both pain and exhaustion are the two main symptoms of FMS. These symptoms are thought to be a result of a hyperactive sympathetic nervous system which produces too much epinephrine and norepinepherine, causing it to go into "overdrive." This overdrive leaves the body depleted. FMS sometimes occurs after an ordinary infection (bacterial or viral) or trauma, such as whiplash from an auto accident. Because of this FMS has been compared to reflex sympathetic dystrophy (RSD), explained earlier in this chapter as a condition that can develop after trauma. Simply, the body's immune defense system is abnormal and patients don't fight infection and stress or heal as they should, resulting in exaggerated chronic and widespread pain.

Patients with FMS experience a variety of symptoms including widespread pain, fatigue, stiffness, fragmented sleep and sleep disorders, poor memory and concentration, slowed reading and information processing, hypermobility of the joints (they are double-jointed, which may make them more vulnerable to injury), vision and balance problems (vestibular disorder), reduced muscle coordination, sub-normal body temperature, headaches and sensitivity to light, sound, cold and/or heat, skin rashes, chest pain, a feeling of bladder fullness, irritable bladder, and they can have IC/BPS. Dan Clauw, M.D., director of the University of Michigan's FM (fibromyalgia) research team, has worked with an ophthalmologist to prove that people who have dry and itchy eyes, but still test normally, have the regional equivalent of FMS (i.e. interstitial cystitis or IBS) of the eyes. Clauw explains that "This disease (FMS) spares no area of the body, which only makes sense because we get sensory input from everywhere in the body." Like IC/BPS, FMS can be genetic and is often accompanied by other conditions, such as temporomandibular disorder, restless leg syndrome, mitral valve prolapse, and hypothyroidism. Although a diagnosis of IC/BPS does not indicate a diagnosis of another condition, IC/BPS patients, especially those with FMS, may experience overlapping conditions.

Since sleep deprivation is a main symptom, a variety of medications are used to increase the levels of serotonin, norepineph-erine, and dopamine in FMS patients. Some of the medications are also used for IC/BPS and CP/CPPS, such as amitriptyline, Neurontin, and Lyrica. Selective serotonin and norepinephrine reuptake inhibitors (SSNRIs), like Cymbalta (duloxetine), are also used for FMS, but are often not tolerated by IC/BPS patients. (Some IC/BPS patients may experience bladder symptoms with Cymbalta due to increased urinary retention.) Although both Lyrica and Cymbalta are approved for FMS by the FDA, patients usually require multiple medications and therapies to calm the sympathetic nervous system, including alternative therapies, supplements (especially Omega 3), and the right type of exercise. *Refer to Chapters Three and Four.*

Research has shown that the lack of quality sleep in FMS patients triggers more pain and sometimes depression. According to Silvia Bigatti, Ph.D., "Depression may be the end result of a process that begins with sleep problems." The FMS patient's mood is affected by the type of sleep deprivation that impairs physical functioning.

Similar to IC/BPS, FMS can be diagnosed through a process of exclusion; however, a rheumatologist can perform an examination to detect sensitive "tender points" in certain areas of the body. These tender points cluster around the neck, shoulders, chest, hips, knees, and elbows and are considered the hallmark of FMS. A patient must have at least 11 of the 18 tender points to meet the FMS criteria. Patients with FMS also experience trigger points. Some experts believe that the tender points are simply trigger points.

Most tender points in FMS patients are located in the neck and shoulders. The major sympathetic ganglia network (of nerves) is located in this area.

Chronic fatigue syndrome/myalgic encephalomyelitis (CFS/ME)

CFS/ME is finally recognized as a real condition instead of a psychiatric disorder. CFS/ME affects at least 17 million people worldwide and the rate of CFS/ME in the IC/BPS population is high. CFS also overlaps FMS and is sometimes considered to be the same condition. CFS/ME patients appear to have abnormalities in the immune system, the brain, and the autonomic and endocrine systems. Symptoms, perhaps some caused by cystokines (substances that are secreted by immune cells in the body, including the central nervous system), include fragmented sleep, exhaustion, cognitive and memory problems, IBS, pelvic pain, brain fog, and flu-like body aches, as well as tender lymph nodes and sore throats. CFS/ME patients are also likely to have hypermobile joints, as well as IBS, allergies, multiple chemical sensitivity (MCS), endometriosis, and other disorders. Men with CFS/ME appear to have a higher rate of chronic prostatitis/chronic pelvic pain syndrome (CP/CPPS) than men without CFS/ME. As with most other chronic conditions, patients must have symptoms six months or more for a diagnosis.

Chronic fatigue is not the same as chronic fatigue syndrome.

In the past, CFS/ME was blamed on the Epstein-Barr virus. Although some patients do have one or more herpes virus infections (such as Epstein-Barr virus), and seem to respond well to the antiviral drug Valtrex (valacyclovir hydrochloride), Epstein-Barr is no longer considered the culprit. In recent years, researchers have identified a retrovirus named xenotropic murine leukemia virus (XMRV), which is in the same family of viruses as AIDS and may have the ability to activate other viruses. Researchers have not yet proven that the virus causes CFS/ME because patients are prone to health problems anyway, and may just be vulnerable to the virus. Some researchers are trying to establish CFS/ME as an infectious disease. Still, trials on antiviral drugs with patients are underway in several countries.

Typical treatments for CFS/ME are aimed at restoring sleep and normal blood pressure, treating infections and allergies, improving nutrition, and participating in some gentle exercise to help to relieve joint and muscle pain.

Temporomandibular Disorder (TMJD)

TMJD (or TMD) is a joint dysfunction of the jaw that causes severe jaw, face, head, ear, neck, and shoulder pain, migraines, vision problems, and dizziness. The syndrome is genetic, influenced by hormones, and caused by the muscles and ligaments around the jaw and not the jaw joint itself. Denniz Zolnoun, M.D., of the University of North Carolina in Chapel Hill, compares the jaw to the pelvic area. She notes that both areas have multiple muscles and are equally complicated. A high number of her patients with vulvar vestibulitis syndrome complain of orofacial pain.

Experts believe that TMJD does not typically exist on its own. It typically co-occurs with regional and widespread pain conditions such as IBS, FMS, CFS, vulvodynia, and IC/BPS. Patients with autoimmune disorders, such as Lupus and rheumatoid arthritis may also experience this syndrome. It takes an average of four years to get a proper diagnosis and patients may need a team of doctors including a neurologist, a rheumatologist, and a pain management doctor. Drugs used to treat TMJD are often the same ones that treat the overlapping conditions. Cymbalta has been studied for its effectiveness.

Releasing trigger points in the sternocleidomastoid muscle of the neck is usually necessary to relieve the accumulated tension in the jaw.

Migraine Headaches

Serious headaches are triggered by an event which causes hyper-excitement of the cell membranes around the brain. The excitement causes the trigeminal nerve (which supplies the muscles of the head and face) to become irritated. The irritation, in turn, causes the brain to produce throbbing pain, as well as other symptoms, such as light and sound sensitivity, dizziness, and nausea. Straining, coughing, and leaning over can worsen the pain. When a migraine is only on one side, it is often due to trigger points on that side. Some experts believe that trigger points in the neck and head are responsible for irritating the trigeminal nerve.

In Chinese medicine, the area of a headache indicates an involved organ. An interesting example is pain that occurs in the back of the head. This type of headache is an indication of a bladder problem in Chinese medicine. When this is the case, the bladder would be treated to relieve the pain in the back of the head.

Serious headaches are common in both IC/BPS and CP/CPPS patients, but they affect more women than men. This is probably due to hormonal fluctuations. Women often experience pre-menstrual migraines. Serious headaches in the IC/BPS and CP/CPPS population are usually either chronic or migraine. The medications used for serious headaches are often the same ones that help relieve bladder symptoms, including Elavil (amitriptyline) and Valium (diazepam). Some selective serotonin reuptake inhibitors (SSRIs), such as Prozac (fluoxetine), are also used for migraines, but many of the SSRIs irritate the bladder. The fact that trigger points are common in both IC/BPS and FMS means that patients need to address their trigger points for relief, as well as prevention. Trigger-point therapy can be done by a therapist, a partner, or by oneself. *See Chapter Four.*

Diet also plays a role in serious headaches. Many of the same foods that exasperate IC/BPS symptoms also trigger migraines in susceptible people. Aged foods, smoked foods, and foods and drinks high in histamine, such as red wine, are all on the "foods to avoid list" for migraine patients.

Patients who have multiple chemical sensitivity (MCS) may suffer with sinus migraines. Trigger point therapy on the face, head, neck, and shoulders can help to release the tension caused by noxious odors and chemicals. Obviously, these types of headaches require environmental changes. (Refer to Chapter Six.)

Sjögren's Syndrome (SS)

IC/BPS can occur in association with Sjögren's syndrome, also called Sicca Syndrome. This autoimmune disease attacks both the collagen and the secretary glands of the body. The two areas most affected are the tear ducts and the salivary glands of the mouth. Symptoms include dry and burning eyes and mouth, as well as vaginal dryness in females. These symptoms make treatment difficult for patients with overlapping conditions such as IC/BPS and FMS. Medications, such as anticholinergics and other medications that have drying side effects, are particularly irritating to patients with SS. Patients may do best with a good pain specialist who understands their sensitivity to medications and their need for pain relief.

There seems to be a connection with SS and IC/BPS, IBS, and inflammatory bowel disease (IBD). The mucous membranes are affected in all of these conditions, and permeability, especially in the bladder and intestine wall, may be responsible for an immune response. The fact that a number of IC/BPS patients also have SS, Lupus, and IBD (Crohn's disease and ulcerative colitis) points to an immune system involvement.

Chronic Prostatitis/Chronic Pelvic Pain Syndrome (CP/CPPS)

CP/CPPS is an abnormal sensory condition that causes chronic pelvic pain and urinary symptoms in men. Since there is no abnormal influence on the prostrate, the National Institutes of Health (NIH) diagnostic classifications renamed the condition chronic pelvic pain syndrome (CPPS) for research purposes.

Patients are usually diagnosed with chronic abacterial prostatitis when they see a doctor for painful urinary symptoms and show no signs of an infection (infection can co-exist with CP/CPPS in some instances). Like IC/BPS in men, CP/CPPS can cause pain in the perineum, scrotum, groin, penis, rectum, and abdomen but mostly perineal and ejaculatory pain. Unlike IC/BPS, there is no anti-proliferative (APF) found in their urine, and their frequency and urgency may be less severe. However, a majority of the CP/CPPS population have bladders that appear the same as IC/BPS upon cystoscopy with hydrodystention. And although CP/CPPS is not the same condition as IC/BPS, the two conditions may be different variants or manifestations of the same disease, and may have a possible genetic relationship. As mentioned before, these two conditions can co-exist. Like other chronic pain patients, some CP/CPPS patients may benefit from tricyclic antidepressants, antispasmodics, and drugs like Neurontin and Lyrica. Neurontin and other drugs used to treat migraines are sometimes used to treat ejaculation pain.

Allergies

Mast cells release histamines that cause inflammation and pain during an allergic reaction to an allergen. Increased numbers of mast cells are found in the bladder wall of IC/BPS patients. Many patients suffer with allergies and test positive for IgE production. (IgE plays a role in allergy.) Because mast cells (in humans) have estrogen receptors, many women with IC/BPS may experience flare-ups when their estrogen levels are highest. Cromolyn sodium (Gastrocrom and Nasalcrom) might be helpful to fight allergies, including food allergies. Cromolyn sodium has also been known to calm IC/BPS symptoms in some patients. All patients taking antihistamines for allergies and/or to reduce the high number of mast cells in their bladder walls must avoid decongestants.

Panic Disorder

Panic disorder causes sudden feelings of fear, as well as shortness of breath and heart palpitations. Although these symptoms make panic disorder sound like a psychological problem, this disorder is actually linked to several conditions. Patients with hypo-thyroidism, mitral valve prolapse, allergies, migraines, and other overlapping conditions, such as IC/BPS, CP/CPPS, FMS, and CFS/ME may suffer with panic disorder. These relationships point to a problem in the central nervous system, as well as a genetic link. A good example is the IC/BPS patient who has one child with IC/BPS and another child with only panic disorder. Medications prescribed for panic disorder include Elavil and Valium.

Pudendal Neuralgia

Pudendal neuralgia (PN) is inflammation of the pudendal nerve. The pudendal nerve begins in the sacral roots and crosses the piriformis muscle (a hip rotator). The perineal branch of the pudendal nerve supplies the muscles of the pelvic floor, the labial and scrotal skin, and the clitoral and penile erectile functions. The symptoms of PN, which are similar and sometimes mistaken for IC/BPS, include pelvic pain, urgency, and frequency, difficulty with urination and defecation, and painful intercourse. Pain in women may affect the urethra, vulva, perineum (the area be-tween the vagina and anus in women and between the scrotum and anus in men), and buttocks. Pain in men occurs in the penis, urethra, perineum, scrotum, and buttocks and can be felt with ejaculation. Because the perineal area is the most common area of pain, patients are advised to elevate this area while sitting to prevent pressure.

PN can result after childbirth, vaginal surgery, chronic vaginal infections, injury to the tailbone, and compression from a bike seat. Pelvic floor dysfunction (PFD) and sacroiliac problems can also be responsible for an inflamed pudendal nerve. Because sit-ting triggers the pain, patients are more comfortable standing, lying down, or sitting on a toilet seat (which relieves the pain because there is no pressure on the perineum).

A variety of medications can be used in nerve blocks to treat PN, such as an injection of an anesthetic, a steroid, a benzodiaz-epine, an opioid, BCG (which is controversial), heparin (which must *not* contain alcohol or phenol), or epinephrine. Because PN can co-exist with IC/BPS, epinephrine may not be a good choice for patients. Epinephrine is a known IC/BPS trigger. When a block only works temporarily, the patient can be tested to see if the nerve is entrapped. If it is, a patient has a choice of surgery or nerve stimulation, but it's necessary to find an expert in the field, because surgery is not always reliable. However, the sooner the pain is addressed, the less chance that central sensitization will occur.

Autoimmune Diseases and IC/BPS

Many doctors who are familiar with IC/BPS patients agree the condition has an immune system involvement. The fact that there is a high prevalence of allergies in patients suggests that IC/BPS may be caused by a compromised immune system. There's also the fact that many autoimmune diseases impact the IC/BPS population more than the general population. The most common overlapping autoimmune diseases include Sjögren's syndrome (previously discussed), Lupus, which affects the skin, the joints and vital organs, and inflammatory bowel disease, which involves either ulcerative colitis or Crohn's disease. There are even some IC/BPS patients *without* an autoimmune disease who test positive or borderline for certain antibodies and factors that indicate an autoimmune process in the body.

A large percentage of female IC/BPS patients are diagnosed with endometriosis and/or vulvodynia. These conditions will be discussed in Chapter Eight.

Resources

Associations, Foundations, and Networks

Interstitial Cystitis/Bladder Pain Syndrome (IC/BPS) and Chronic Prostatitis/Chronic Prostatitis Pain Syndrome (CP/CPPS)

Interstitial Cystitis Association (ICA)
www.ichelp.org • (703) 442-2070

Interstitial Cystitis Network
www.ic-network.com• (707) 538-9442

P.U.R.E.H.O.P.E. (Pelvic Urological Resources and Education Helping Others with Pelvic Pain Everywhere)
www.pure-hope.org • (281) 500-4656

National Kidney and Urologic Diseases Information Clearinghouse (NKUDIC)
www.kidney.niddk.nih.gov • (800) 891-5390

American Foundation for Urologic Disease (AFUD)
www.afud.org • (800) 828-7866

American Urologic Association (AUAF)
www.urologyhealth.org • (800) 828-7866

Prostatitis Foundation (PF)
www.prostatitis.org • (309) 325-7184
(613) 548-7832 (Canada)• Information packet (800) 891-4200

International Pelvic Pain Society (IPPS)
www.pelvicpain.org • (847) 517-8712

Irritable Bowel Syndrome (IBS)

International Foundation for Functional Gastrointestinal Disorders (IFFGD)
www.iffgd.org • (888) 964-2001

National Digestive Diseases Information Clearinghouse
www.digestive.niddk.nih.gov • (800) 891-5389

Fibromyalgia (FMS) and Chronic Fatigue Syndrome (CFIDS)

CFIDS Association of America
www.cfids.org • (704) 365-2343

American Fibromyalgia Syndrome Association (AFSA)
www.afsafund.org • (520) 733-1570

National Fibromyalgia Association
www.fmaware.org • (714) 921-0150

Tempomandibular Joint Dysfunction (TMJ)

TMJ Association (TMJA)
www.tmj.org • (262) 432-0350

Migraine Headaches

The National Migraine Association (MAGNUM)
www.migraines.org • (703) 340-1929

Sjögren's Syndrome

National Sjögren's Syndrome Association (NASSA)
www.sjogrenssyndrome.org • (800) 395-NSSA (6772)

Sjögren's Syndrome Foundation
www.sjogrens.org • (800) 475-6473

Allergies

Asthma and Allergy Foundation of America (AAFA)
www.aafa.org • (800) 727-8462 (7-ASTHMA)

Panic Disorder

Anxiety Disorder Association of America (ADAA)
www.adaa.org • (240) 485-1001

Pudendal Neuralgia (PN)

Society for Pudendal Neuralgia (SPuN)
www.oswego.edu/~msheppar/isc325/spuninfo
(315) 312-2500 (SUNY Oswego)

Natural Supplements

CystoProtek
www.cysto-protek.com • (855) 874-0970 (information)
(800) 328-0503 (orders)

ProstaProtek
www.algonot.com • (800) 254-6668

Cysta-Q and Prosta-Q
www.cystaq.com • (877) 284-3976

Prelief
www.prelief.com • (800) 994.4711

Desert Harvest Aloe Vera
www.desertharvest.com • (800) 222-3901

Books

Interstitial Cystitis Survival Guide, Robert M. Moldwin, M.D., F.A.C.S.

Headache in the Pelvis, David Wise, Ph.D.

Interstitial Cystitis, Grannum R. Sant, M.D.

Chapter Two

FOLLOWING A DIET FOR IC/BPS

Today, most urologists who treat IC/BPS and CP/CPPS patients understand and accept that diet plays a vital role in the treatment of these conditions. But this has not always been the case. Not too long ago many urologists, as well as IC/BPS researchers, either did not acknowledge (due to a lack of scientific evidence) or even know about the diet for IC/BPS. Thankfully, things began to change in 2000 when IC/BPS advocate, Robert Moldwin, M.D., director of the Interstitial Cystitis Center in Long Island, N.Y., legitimized the IC diet in his book *The Interstitial Cystitis Survival Guide.* Even so, there still remained skeptics who were not listening to their patients or acknowledging the lists of "foods to avoid." Dr. Moldwin and Barbara Shorter, Ed.D., R.D., C.D.N., worked to further prove the effects of certain foods on the IC/BPS bladder. The results of their joint study were presented at the American Urological Association (AUA) annual meeting in 2006. The following year their study appeared in the *Journal of Urology.* Dr. Moldwin confirmed the importance of the IC diet once again.

Other experts climbed on board during these years. In 2004 Jill Osborne, M.A., President and Founder of the IC Network, Bev Laumann, author of *A Taste of the Good Life: A Cookbook for an Interstitial Cystitis Diet,* Julie Beyer, M.A., R.D., author of the *Confident Choices* series, Barbara Gordon, R.D., former Executive Director of the ICA along with Barbara Shorter decided to do a diet survey. The results of their survey overwhelmingly supported the diet; the majority of patients said that the IC diet absolutely helped them to prevent symptoms. Because of these efforts the AUA now recognizes the diet as one of the initial treatments for the symptoms of IC/BPS.

So why do certain foods, drinks, and ingredients irritate patients' bladders? In 1998 IC/BPS patient and author Bev Laumann explained in her book, *A Taste of the Good Life: A Cookbook for an Interstitial Cystitis Diet,* how certain foods send messages within the nervous system and trigger symptoms. These foods contain the monamines tyramine and histamine (which are neurotransmitters), as well as the amino acids tyrosine, tryptophan, and phenylalanine (which are also chemical messengers). The monamines tyramine and histamine appear to be the most irritating offenders. Foods containing these different compounds are also known to trigger pain in people with irritable bowel syndrome (IBS) and migraine headaches.

Laumann studied different IC diet lists and comprised her own list of problem foods. Laumann's list of "foods to avoid" remains the easiest and safest approach to detecting irritating foods, because it closely follows the basic guidelines. To discover which foods irritate your bladder, eliminate all of the foods on the following list. If your bladder symptoms calm down after a few weeks, or a month, introduce *one* food at a time. This process of elimination is the only way to determine which foods sensitize your bladder. (It's also important to avoid new therapies during this process.)

Group 1 Foods (Foods To Be Avoided)

aged cheeses (i.e., cheddar, Swiss, gouda, Roquefort, brie)
aged, processed, cured, and smoked meats and fish (or any animal product with nitrates)
anchovies
apples
apricots
aspartame (i.e., Nutrasweet)
avocados
bananas
beer
berries (except blueberries and blackberries)
caffeine

cantaloupes
carbonated drinks
caviar
cherries (sweet and sour)
chicken livers
chocolate
chutney
citric acid
citrus fruit and citrus juices
coffee
corned beef
cranberries and cranberry juice
eggplant
fava beans
grapes
green tea
hot spices: cayenne, chiles and chile powder, cloves, cumin,
    curry powder, fenugreek, and paprika
lima beans
mayonnaise
miso
MSG (monosodium glutamate)
nectarines
peaches
pineapples
plums
pomegranates
raw globe or green onions
red wine
rhubarb
rye and sourdough bread
saccharine
salad dressing (commercially prepared)
sodium benzoate or potassium benzoate
soy sauce (except some low-sodium)
strawberries
tamari sauce
tea

tofu
tomatoes
vinegar
white wine and other alcoholic beverages when not cooked
yogurt

Many patients and dieticians are under the misconception that balancing the acid/alkaline levels in the body can help to control the symptoms of IC/BPS, but this is not so. Acidic-tasting foods that turn alkaline in the system can still end up flaring the IC/BPS bladder.

Group 2 Foods (Limited-Use Foods That *May* Be Bladder-Safe When Used In Small Amounts)

cooking sherry
cooked globe onions, cooked green onions, raw chives in
     very small amounts
low-sodium soy sauce
nuts (other than almonds, pine nuts, and cashews)
preservatives and artificial ingredients (this does not
     include artificial sweeteners)
ripe blackberries
bananas
white chocolate
dried cranberries
raisins
herb teas
yogurt, including frozen yogurt

Giving up favorite foods can feel like giving up little parts of yourself. There's a saying, "You can't let go until you find a replacement." Although there are alternatives and substitutes, each patient has a unique tolerance for different foods. Trying a new food, even if it is considered "safe," may not work for you. New patients just discovering their diet restrictions may have to learn through "trial by error." Therefore, using moderation and limiting new foods to times when your bladder symptoms are stable is not only essential to avoid a flare-up, but also necessary to distinguish if a food is really an irritant.

Occasionally, patients who have been on the IC diet for a good period of time and have been treated for symptoms, discover they can tolerate foods which they could not before. This can also work in reverse. Sometimes a food that has been completely safe can all of a sudden become irritating to the bladder. Reintroducing it later may work out or the food may always have to be avoided. The bladder can change and so can the body's chemistry. IC/BPS is full of surprises, for better or worse. Taking control of your diet can help to reduce the unwanted surprises.

The following dietary alternatives and suggestions have been collected from the broad and individual experiences of many different IC/BPS patients. They should be tried in moderation, *one food* at a time, when bladder symptoms are stable.

Fruit

Pears are considered the most bladder-safe fruit. But pears are among foods found to be highly affected by pesticides. To avoid neurotoxic pesticide residue, buy organic pears and pear juice. Always avoid pears packed in artificial sweetener, and pears that are badly bruised. They may be in the process of fermentation, which may affect the bladder.

Pear juice from the health food store and/or pear juice made for babies, such as Gerber's, may be bladder-safe, but some patients may need to dilute the juice with water. It's important to avoid pear juice that is mixed with other fruit and/or contains citric acid. If tolerated, pure pear juice adds a lot of flavor to cooked dishes.

Other fruits to try one at a time are: **honeydew** and **watermelon, blueberries,** and **blackberries.** Pure blueberry juice (usually a concentrate which you add to water) and Minute Maid's reduced-acid Orange Juice agree with many patients, but, again, tolerance is very individual. Blueberries are usually tolerated and provide super antioxidants that protect cell life. Another benefit of these berries is they act just as cranberries do to prevent urinary tract infections (UTIs). Always check soups and cereals found at health food stores for added fruit juice that is not bladder-safe.

Tomatoes are typically irritating to the IC/BPS bladder. For some patients even yellow tomatoes and Creoles (true Creole tomatoes are only grown in Louisiana) are not safe. Patients who can eat tomatoes may do best with the hothouse variety and not the commercial tomatoes found in large groceries. Canned tomatoes, tomato pastes, sauces, and juices are naturally high in acid, and many also contain the bladder irritant citric acid. When tolerated, a teaspoon of pure tomato sauce without citric acid can be added to certain cooked dishes to provide tomato flavor. This includes bladder-safe chicken or beef broth for those who miss tomato soup, which usually contains citric acid and other irritants.

Some brands of tomato pastes and sauces may contain citric acid and not list it in their ingredients. To find the safest sauces contact manufacturers. Tomato products containing "natural flavor" may also contain citric acid and other bladder irritants.

Patients who miss the taste of **lemons** can substitute this citrus fruit with herbs such as lemon thyme, lemon balm, lemon grass, and Thai basil. These herbs are usually tolerated in cooked dishes. Of course, Minute Maid low-acid Orange Juice also provides citrus flavor to certain dishes. Be aware that other brands of low acid orange juice may contain citric acid.

Nuts

Nuts provide high-energy and nutritious snacks. Nuts are full of protein, fiber, vitamins, calcium, and other minerals, as well as healthful fats. IC/BPS patients seem to tolerate almonds and cashews the best, but they may also find peanuts and walnuts agreeable. Walnuts are rich in Omega 3 fatty acids, which help prevent inflammatory diseases. Chopped walnuts, sprinkled over oatmeal, make a nutritious breakfast or snack. Nut and seed butters (such as almond, cashew, and sunflower seed butter) are also very healthy, and also make a good breakfast when spread on a piece of toast or a rice cake and eaten with a pear on the side.

Tolerance to nuts is highly individual and some people with allergies may have to avoid nuts. Although almonds appear to be the most bladder-friendly, it's worth experimenting with various nuts, if you are not allergic. (Some patients find they can drink almond milk. Although it is very healthful, not all patients can tolerate it.)

Coffee and Tea

IC/BPS patients who can drink a *little* coffee, either with caffeine or decaffeinated, may want to try a dark roast. Contrary to what most people think, dark roast coffee beans are the lowest in caffeine and acid. Drinking drip coffee is another way to avoid high acidity. Dripping coffee through a paper filter not only lowers acidity, it also helps to remove pesticide residue. (Coffee and cotton are the two most heavily sprayed crops.) When using a cone drip system wait 20 seconds after the water boils before pouring it over the coffee. Doing this will further reduce the acidity.

Caffeine in decaffeinated coffee should always be removed by a pure water process and not a chemical process. Decaffeinated coffee still contains some caffeine, and coffee in general is a diuretic and will cause frequency.

Like coffee, tea is also acidic. Some patients find low-acid coffee more tolerable than tea. To be on the cautious side, when trying a new tea, dunk the tea bag or tea ball only once or twice in the hot water before drinking.

Sensitive patients can easily determine whether a tea is bladder-safe. But, when a tea passes the bladder test, patients should still only use a few dunks before drinking. Weak tea is usually essential to avoid symptoms, so water should never be poured over a tea bag unless patients are not sensitive. This also applies to herbal teas.

Herbal teas offer many benefits, but some are very powerful and/or acidic, and contain various medicinal properties. Herbal teas can act as diuretics, astringents, antispasmodics, sedatives, stimulants, antiseptics, expectorants, laxatives, and more. Although a good percentage of IC/BPS patients cannot tolerate many herbal teas or must drink very weak tea, one doctor specializing in herbs created a custom tea to relieve IC/BPS symptoms. The tea is made from 12 different herbs. Many of these herbs when used alone can cause side effects. But the combination of these herbs is meant to prevent side effects. The outcome of success for this tea is mixed. When first trying this special tea, use one dunk of the tea bag or ball, take one sip of the tea and then wait to see if you experience a reaction.

Some IC/BPS patients find weak chamomile, marshmallow root, cornsilk, willow bark, mint, and horsetail grass tea tolerable. See Chapter Seven for more information on the alternative uses of herbal teas. To order Dr. Ching-Yao Shi's tea, see Resources at the end of this chapter. Refer to the IC Network for coffee substitutes.

Sweets and Sodas

Caramel and carob seem to replace chocolate for many patients, but chocolate can be very hard to give up. White chocolate, which is usually bladder-safe, does not have the same effect. However, white chocolate can be very satisfying when mixed with hot milk or added to cookies and desserts. When patients crave real chocolate, they can try a very small amount of a quality dark chocolate. Milk chocolate, on the other hand, can irritate the bladder.

Patients who can eat sugar may want to add a little honey to the sweet side of their diet. Honey is a prime source of mineral salts and offers many nutritive benefits (honey should come from a well-known source). Because some honeys tend to be strong, try only a small amount when first testing. Keep in mind that there are many different varieties to choose from. Maple syrup is another option for sweetening and flavor.

Patients who must avoid sugar can try a small amount of Splenda or Truvia (which is a better choice), but all patients should avoid aspartame, which is found in NutraSweet and Equal. The artificial sweetener saccharine must also be avoided to prevent symptoms. These sweeteners are nerve stimulators and begin stimulation on the tongue, then move through the system to the nerves in the bladder. Some preservatives are also nerve stimulators.

Tonic water, soda water, and commercial sodas are typically irritating to the bladder. Carbonation causes frequency and sodas often contain citric acid. Patients can let sodas go flat or add a little salt to get rid of the bubbles to reduce carbonation. Coca-Cola is sometimes tolerable because it doesn't contain citrus fruit. Or a clear soda such as 7-Up is tolerable because it does not contain caffeine and other ingredients found in Coca-Cola. Root Beer (without caffeine) is also well tolerated by some patients, although there are many IC/BPS patients who must avoid all sodas. All patients should avoid diet sodas to prevent symptoms.

Patients prone to yeast infections should limit the amount of sugar in their diets.

Salad Dressings, Condiments, and Seasoning

Eating fresh and raw vegetables is very important, but salad dressings contain a number of bladder irritants. You can replace dressings with olive oil, and mild dry herbs can be added for flavor and nutrients. Olive oil mixed with salt, pepper (some IC/BPS patients must avoid cracked black pepper), and a dash of oregano is wonderful on salad. Garlic powder, salt, pepper, and oregano or dill mixed with olive oil and a touch of honey (if tolerated) also make a good salad dressing. Olive or vegetable oil can also be mixed with plain yogurt and fresh dill for those who can have yogurt.

Olives and olive mixes are very flavorful and can help provide the tart taste associated with the vinegar in salad dressings. However, it's essential to know the ingredients used to brine and preserve the individual type of olive or olives in a mix. Most olives contain vinegar and/or citric acid. Both of which should be avoided. Lactic acid is sometimes used instead to preserve olives and seems to be bladder-friendly for most patients. Look for black Beldies, black Provencal, plain oil cured black olives, Nicoise Coquillos, Picholines, green olives stuffed with pimento, and Mediterranean olive mixes. These are often available with no citric acid or vinegar. Some olive bars in grocery stores list the ingredients in their olives. Be sure to read the labels when buying bottled olives. Bottled Mufallata olive salad and cracked olive salad deliver great taste when added to salads and sandwiches, but vinegar and citric acid may be added to some brands and not listed. Make friends with the olive vendor at your local market and call the manufacturers to double-check ingredients. It's worth it if you like olives.

When cooked, vinegar will somewhat breakdown but citric acid will not. So, a patient has a better chance of tolerating a white pizza with olives that contain vinegar only, than a pizza with olives that contain citric acid. Of course, vinegar is still a known irritant.

Multi-purpose Kenzoil adds flavor to salads, sandwiches, pasta, and other dishes, and can be used as a dipping oil and a marinade. Kenzoil is made with olive oil, basil, garlic, and other seasoning, is free of gluten, dairy, nuts, sugar, and vinegar, and is also Vegan. Olive oil can always be added for patients who want to cut the garlic taste. Kenzoil is found in the refrigerated section in grocery stores and health food stores. Pyramid Herb Seasoning/Mediterranean Salad is a wonderful natural herbal seasoning that is delicious when sprinkled over salad with olive oil. Ingredients include sunflower seeds and a little soya, but this seasoning seems bladder-safe for many. *See Resources.*

Because egg whites can neutralize acidity, a small amount of Hellmann's Real Mayonnaise or Miracle Whip is sometimes tolerated. Mayonnaise can be added to olive oil for flavor in salads and sandwiches. Patients who are sensitive to soy may try Hain's Safflower Mayonaise. (Most mayonnaise contains soy oil.) Patients should steer clear of organic and diet mayonnaises because they usually contain more lemon and vinegar. Softened cream cheese (including the lower fat variety) or butter flavored with herbs can replace mayonnaise products.

Using different oils and wines will put more flavor and nutrition into your diet. A small amount of toasted sesame oil and/or sesame seeds enhances flavor in stir fry, rice, chicken, and egg dishes. Since alcohol evaporates when heated most patients can enjoy a little wine in their cooked foods. One such flavorful wine is Mirin. This cultured sweet rice *wine* is found in health food stores and Asian groceries. Be sure not to mistake rice vinegar for rice wine. Rice vinegar will irritate the bladder.

Dried herbs, such as dill, thyme, basil, marjoram, oregano, bay leaf, parsley, rosemary, sage, and celery salt should be bladder-safe, but try one at a time to determine which can be used. Herbs offer important antioxidant properties. Garlic also offers healthful benefits as well as flavor to foods. Cooked garlic and garlic powder appear to be tolerated by many patients, but raw garlic is too strong for some. Chives, shallots, scallions, and leeks are also part of the garlic family. When cooked, most of these are bladder-safe but patients may have to limit the amount of cooked leeks they consume. Raw onions, including green onions, should be avoided, and patients must be very careful to avoid hidden raw onions in salads. On the other hand, a small amount of cooked onions is usually well tolerated; however, onion powder may be an irritant.

Patients who find cooked onions bladder-friendly may want to eat them routinely. Onions are a good source of quercetin, which reduces allergy symptoms, and is found in some of the supplements suggested for IC/BPS. Onions contain powerful protective and anti-inflammatory properties and are not only healthy, they also add wonderful flavor to stir-fry, eggs, and other cooked dishes. Capers actually offer more quercetin than onions. However, they are usually brined in vinegar. Look for capers in a salt-only brine (which mostly come in a jar, although some Whole Foods Markets list their bulk capers without a vinegar brine). Capers are wonderful in salads, eggs, and stir-fry.

Spicy foods should usually be avoided because they stimulate histamine release and cause pain. Then again, patients who seem to tolerate and enjoy some spicy foods can benefit from trying favorite spices one at a time when symptoms are stable. For instance, a Thai dish consisting of curry, ginger, acidic sauces, and peppers may prove terribly irritating, but the ingredient tumeric (used in curries) alone and/or the ginger alone may be agreeable. Combinations of spices in cooked dishes can make all the difference.

Peppers, like wines, can vary. For example, a small amount of mild paprika may irritate the bladder while a small amount of fine black pepper or cayenne may be benign. Paprika is added to enhance color in many foods, including hot dogs and sausage. It is also in many hamburger and hot dog buns. Of course, not every IC/BPS patient has a reaction to paprika or can tolerate black and/or white pepper, and/or cayenne. Patients need to wear gloves or coat their hands thoroughly with vegetable oil before handling hot peppers, raw onions, or hot dried spices, because they can linger on the hands and transfer to the bladder.

> *IC/BPS patients worried about the strong garlic odor after a DMSO instillation may want to treat "like with like." Everyone in the household has a garlicky meal the day of the treatment. Drinking a glass of whole milk immediately after a DMSO treatment might also help to neutralize the odor.*

Cheese

Aged cheese is high in tyramine and can be very irritating to the IC/BPS bladder, but there are alternatives to fill in its place. One alternative is American cheese, but it may not seem so healthy for those who are used to healthy foods. Other more healthy alternatives include mozzarella and ricotta unless they contain vinegar. Always check the ingredients to avoid a flare-up. Farmer's cheese, fresh Mexican cheese, fresh goat cheese, cottage, and cream cheese are usually bladder-safe. Both feta and mozzarella are wonderful in salads, especially with olives cured only in salt brine. Parmesan cheese in a can is also versatile and sometimes tolerated. But patients with irritable bowel syndrome (IBS) may not tolerate the cellulose used in canned parmesan cheese. Some IC/BPS patients find they can have a little regular parmesan cheese.

> *IC/BPS patients prone to constipation and/or yeast infections should limit their dairy intake. Patients with IBS might consider replacing cow dairy products with goat dairy products which are easier to digest.*

Salt

Patients sensitive to salt may need to avoid foods high in sodium. Bev Laumann has found that salt can be good, bad, or have no effect on the IC/BPS bladder. Several different factors appear to determine the effects of salt in individual patients:

- Daily water consumption
- How much exercise a patient gets
- Whether a patient has mostly frequency or pain
- Whether a patient has sodium-sensitive high blood pressure
- Whether a patient is sensitive to chlorine in water

Another problem with salty foods may be monosodium glutamate or sodium metabisulfite, which are added to many snack foods that are labeled with "natural flavoring." It's best that patients avoid snack foods which list "natural flavoring" in their contents. Patients may also want to replace regular table salt with rock sea salt. Less is needed and it offers valuable trace elements such as magnesium and calcium. On the contrary, table salt is bleached and contains man-made chemical additives that prevent caking. Some people, however, need the iodine that is added to many table salts to prevent goiter, which is a thyroid problem.

Patients should also avoid foods with the word "hydrolyzed" in their ingredients.

Alcohol

Alcohol in general is a bladder irritant, but there are patients who find they can drink a sweet, low-acid, late-harvest dessert wine such as Sauternes, Barsac, Semillon, Gewurztraminer, or late-harvest Riesling. Late-harvest Riesling is usually the most reasonably priced. A small number of patients have found they can drink well-filtered vodka or straight whiskey, even though whiskey is high in histamine. Alcohol is usually tolerated in cooked dishes because it evaporates, but alcoholic drinks mixed with tonic, fruit juice, or soda must usually be avoided. Plain water and ice (watch out for water and ice made from strongly chlorinated water) are the most bladder-proof mixers.

When drinking alcohol, be sure to do so early in the evening, because alcohol before or near bedtime can interfere with deep sleep (repair time) and wake one up when it wears off. Alcohol may also increase symptoms in patients with other conditions such as fibromyalgia (FMS), irritable bowel syndrome (IBS), and multiple chemical sensitivity (MCS). Patients on medications should use caution and follow labels and instructions.

Over time, which includes stable time (when the bladder is calm), patients do learn what does and what does not work. Unfortunately, it's often by accident.

> *The IC diet was extended and renamed the IC/PBS diet in 2004, after the survey. The survey diet was again revised some years later. After patients have pinpointed their diet culprits, they can refer to the ICA and the ICN for the current diet lists. See Resources in Chapter One. To find bladder-safe recipes refer to the books listed in Resources at the end of this chapter.*

Using Prevention and Assertiveness

The following suggestions can help make your life more comfortable, normal and productive:

- BECOME A DETECTIVE when you shop. Read labels carefully to avoid irritating ingredients such as citric or ascorbic acid and vinegar. Watch out for vinegar, which is often added to bread, and preservatives (natural and not), as well as food dyes.
- LEARN TO QUESTION waiters and waitresses. Call ahead or look online if you are not sure of the food served in a particular restaurant. Most restaurants offer plain (not marinated) steak, or chicken, rice, baked potatoes, and bladder-proof salad (without raw onions, radishes, aged cheeses, or certain seasoned croutons). You can ask for olive oil, or whatever oil they have, on the side. Find restaurants where you can enjoy bladder-safe meals in comfort. Be

aware that some ingredients used in some chain restaurants differ from their foods sold in grocery stores because of the added preservatives used for shelf life.

If you're invited to a dinner party, if possible, call the hostess or host well in advance to ask what foods will be served. Gently explain that you have food intolerance because of a medical condition. Ask if it's possible to plan a plate for your self in order to avoid drawing attention to a problem. If this isn't possible, and it is a casual affair, ask if you can bring your own dish to add to the party. Naturally, there will be times when this won't be possible and you will either have to decline or pretend — which is often impossible.

- EXPLAIN TO YOUR DOCTORS that you must follow a diet similar to a patient who takes MAO inhibitors and also has a gastric ulcer. Patients taking MAO inhibitors, which are a class of antidepressant drugs, must avoid foods or beverages that contain tyramine.
- EAT REGULARLY to prevent flare-ups. Eating small amounts of food throughout the day is very therapeutic for the bladder and can also help patients with fibromyalgia, irritable bowel syndrome, and migraine headaches.
- PATIENTS PRONE TO CONSTIPATION should eat first thing in the morning to stimulate bowel activity. A bowl of hot oatmeal, oat bran, rice bran, or another hot cereal eaten between dinner and bedtime can also add to stimulation the next morning. Eating protein for breakfast is important for stamina and fresh vegetables should be substituted for the lack of fruit in the IC/BPS diet. However, eating a pear a day works as well as eating an apple a day.
- AVOID DEHYDRATION to avoid IC/BPS symptoms. Patients who drink less water have more concentrated urine which can cause pain and frequency, especially in those who have permeable or "leaky bladders" (about 70 percent of IC/BPS patients).
- DRINKING WATER VARIES. Tap water can trigger symptoms due to high levels of chlorine and chemicals. Some patients benefit from using a water filter and some patients

prefer using filtered water for cooking and use bottled water for drinking.

Filtered tap water can also expose patients to chemicals, and tolerance for the various bottled waters is very individual. Bottled water is usually disinfected with ozone and a small number of people, especially those with an autoimmune disease, cannot tolerate ozone. Ozone can be detected with O3 paper from a lab supply company. It also can be removed from water by boiling or exposing it to air. Imported bottled water such as Evian has a long shelf life and, therefore, is usually free of ozone.

Different brands of bottled water also vary as far as tolerance. What one patient can drink, another cannot. IC/BPS patients who experience problems with bottled water may need to drink distilled water instead. Distilled water is sometimes the safest for sensitive IC/BPS patients and can be helpful during a flare-up, but patients who drink bottled water may benefit. This is because distilled water can flush important minerals from your body and should be avoided when ill or dehydrated. Reserving distilled water for flare-ups or alternating it with compatible bottled water may be best. Flavored water and water infused with vitamins should be avoided, although some patients seem to do okay with Dasani, which is infused with minerals.

- PAY ATTENTION TO YOUR HORMONAL CYCLE, because bladder pain, pressure, and frequency can fluctuate with a woman's menstrual cycle. It's important to recognize foods that may be more tolerable during the different times of the menstrual cycle.

  Some female patients discover they can cheat on their IC/BPS diet when their estrogen level is highest, because estrogen helps with the formation of the protective layer of the bladder surface. However, other patients find that, when their estrogen levels are highest, they suffer with IC/BPS symptoms because of the stimulation of mast-cell secretion in their bladders.

- NEUTRALIZE ACIDIC FOODS with the dietary supplement Prelief. Prelief can help relieve burning symptoms.

It can also help patients tolerate a number of foods when taken before or with foods or drinks, and may be used as a calcium-source supplement. You can find Prelief in grocery and drug stores.

Prelief, Tums, baking soda, Tagamet, and Zantac can all be used to neutralize acid; however, patients must consult their doctors or pharmacists before trying these products and medications. They may react unfavorably with medications and/or be dangerous for patients with certain medical conditions.

- CONSULTING A NUTRITIONIST OR DIETITIAN is helpful only if she or he understands IC/BPS or is open to working with the IC/BPS diet. Patients seeing a new dietitian or a nutritionist should bring along a copy of Bev Laumann's *A Taste of the Good Life* and/or Julie Beyer's *Interstitial Cystitis: A Guide for Nutrition Educators.* "Dietary professionals are used to building their patients' immune systems with fruit juices, fortified foods, and vitamins," explains a Philadelphia dietitian who is experienced with IC/BPS. (Experts disagree as to whether the IC/BPS patient's immune system should be boosted or not.) "However, with the diet for IC, most patients have an opportunity to reduce the inflammatory process in their bladders and, therefore, improve their health." She continues, "Because IC/BPS patients are all so different, it can be difficult to determine irritants. Some patients experience pain and frequency soon after their saliva mixes with the juices of an irritant. Others may have a hard time pinpointing the culprit."

- BE AWARE THAT REACTIONS TO VITAMINS AND SUPPLEMENTS aren't well documented. Like a diet for IC/BPS, advice and information should be referred to as a suggested guideline. Also, similar to when trying different foods, patients may need to use caution when trying supplements.

  For instance, vitamins B and C wash through the body and end up in the bladder where they can cause burning, pain, and spasms. Oil soluble vitamins A, D, and E store up in the body rather than washing through to the bladder, so they may be more tolerable. Unfortunately, there are patients who cannot tolerate any vitamins, fortifying supplements, or supplementary oils. Sometimes this is due to the "inert ingredients:" fillers, capsules, binders, and stablizers used in the supplements.

If you cannot take vitamins, put a lot of color into your diet and eat foods rich in vitamins and minerals. Nutritious food is vital to prevent illnesses that can require irritating medications. Broccoli, green, red and yellow peppers, Brussel sprouts, dark leafy vegetables, cabbage, potatoes, and watermelon (if tolerated) contain vitamin C. Vitamin B is found in salmon, tuna, eggs, beef, oysters, pork, milk, mushrooms, broccoli, spinach, dried beans, enriched breads and cereals, brown or enriched rice, and other enriched products (if tolerated).

Irritable Bowel Syndrome (IBS) and Gluten Sensitivity

IBS is common in both IC/BPS and fibromyalgia (FMS) patients. In some countries doctors believe that IBS is celiac disease, a serious condition in which the body has an immune system reaction to gluten. (The reaction causes inflammation in the small intestine.) Other doctors believe that many patients with IBS may actually have *gluten sensitivity* and not celiac disease. Alessio Fasano, M.D., medical director of the University of Maryland Center for Celiac Research, believes that gluten sensitivity actually affects considerably more people than celiac disease. Although not considered serious like celiac, the body's immune system also reacts to grains containing gluten in people with gluten sensitivity.

Gluten is a protein which is actually difficult for all humans to digest. It is found in the grains: wheat, barley, rye, and spelt. Oats are also problematic because they may cross-pollinate with gluten grains or they may be manufactured with the same machinery as other gluten containing grains. (Look for oatmeal labeled gluten-free.) Gluten is also found in the following labeling: "natural flavor," "artificial colors," "modified food starch," and "malt." Fillers in sausages, hot dogs, and deli meats may contain gluten. So may sauces, soups, gravies, and marinades. Beer is brewed with grains that contain gluten. Even medications can contain gluten, labeled as wheat starch, and also some lipsticks. Grains that do not contain gluten are quinoa, buckwheat, and millet. Quinoa and buckwheat are really seeds.

A few tests are available to detect gluten sensitivity. Blood can be drawn to see if IgA and/or IgG antigliadin antibodies are elevated, or the Enterolab gluten sensitivity stool test can be used. The stool test was developed by a doctor who was frustrated by the fact that the blood test doesn't always detect gluten sensitivity. (The test can be ordered online.)

If you suffer with IBS and suspect that you might have a problem with gluten, you can easily detect sensitivity by eliminating gluten from your diet. If your IBS symptoms improve, then you may want to permanently cut gluten foods from your diet. You'll be happily surprised how well you will feel without this culprit. Some IC/BPS patients find that gluten and/or wheat, especially whole wheat, irritates their bladders. There are patients who have reported remission of their IC/BPS symptoms after eliminating gluten. This is not to say that you shouldn't be tested for celiac disease if you suffer with severe IBS symptoms, are losing weight, or have a family member with celiac disease.

> *Many restaurants now offer gluten-free dishes, such as Chinese food made with naturally brewed, wheat-free soy sauce and wheat-free Italian pasta and pizza. (Refer to glutenfreerestaurants.org.) Because gluten is used abundantly in processed, packaged, canned, and frozen foods, more and more grocery stores are offering gluten-free foods. (To learn more, refer to enjoyingglutenfreelife.com.)*

Leaky Gut

A number of IC/BPS and FMS patients experience "leaky gut." Leaky gut is likened to a "leaky bladder." When the intestinal lining becomes too porous, bacteria and other substances enter the intestinal wall causing inflammation and an increase of cytokines (which cause pain). Some experts believe that exposure to these substances also triggers the immune system, because a great number of patients have allergies and sensitivities to foods and medicines. Probiotics appear to help people with leaky gut. *Probiotics will be discussed in Chapter Five.*

Diet and FMS

Unlike the diet for IC/BPS, which eliminates foods and drinks that interfere with bladder function and cause pressure and/or pain, the diet most often recommended for FMS focuses on rotation and elimination of foods that contribute to a constellation of FMS symptoms, such as sleep disturbance, headaches, fatigue, hypoglycemia, skin rashes, gastrointestinal problems, yeast infections, sinus congestion, and more. The foods responsible for these symptoms include:

- **Dairy Products,** which can lead to sinus and gastrointestinal problems, as well as yeast infections
- **Carbohydrates, Sugar, and Fructose,** which are known to promote low blood sugar and yeast infections
- **Saturated Fats,** which can promote inflammation
- **Nightshade Plants** (potatoes, tomatoes, peppers, and eggplant), which also promote inflammation
- **Nerve Stimulators**, such as aspartame (NutraSweet)
- **Flavor Enhancers** (like MSG) and **Preservatives,** all of which affect the nervous system

Nerve stimulators, flavor enhancers, and some preservatives are also referred to as "excitotoxins."

It's not unusual for FMS patients to also have allergies or sensitivities to soy, nuts, wheat, eggs, caffeine, and/or alcohol. FMS patients are encouraged to take vitamins, minerals, and supplements to help calm and control their symptoms. Patients are also advised to avoid cooking processes that diminish important properties in foods, as well as filtered drinking water which depletes natural minerals.

According to Yasemin Turan, M.D., zinc and magnesium are helpful in preventing muscle tenderness and fatigue in FMS patients, yet patients should be aware that these supplements can interfere with thyroid medication. Omega 3 is also considered helpful. Refer to Food-allergy.org for more information on food allergies and intolerances, but keep in mind that many supplements recommended for FMS are irritating to the IC/BPS bladder.

The IC/BPS diet alone can easily overwhelm a new patient. This is why IC/BPS patients, who are also affected by FMS and other conditions, should focus on the IC/BPS diet before experimenting with diets for FMS and IBS (unless their FMS is worse than their IC/BPS, or they have a severe allergy or celiac disease). Realistically, many patients need to tame their bladders first. When their bladder symptoms calm down, they then can try a diet for FMS or another condition if they like.

All patients with FMS and IBS should undergo food allergy testing.

Children with IC/BPS and IBS

Parents need to give their child with IC/BPS and IBS a lot of support, especially regarding diet restrictions. Parents must be willing to research which foods to avoid, experiment with their child's diet, and learn to be very creative. Children usually like the challenge of trying delicious new recipes, eating healthy foods (including fruits and vegetables not treated with pesticides), and learning to read labels. Children are also motivated to learn when they feel special. Parents can reinforce a child who is trying a diet for IC/BPS by taking an interest. Educating family members, the child's school, and the parents of her or his friends are also important.

The most difficult foods for children to exclude are popular snack foods and sweets, especially those containing citric acid and wheat. Referring to Laumann's recipes can be a big help.

Older children may feel resentful, but if certain foods cause them to have painful symptoms, they will most likely decide to avoid these foods. However, there are more issues to deal with for a teen with IC/BPS. Sometimes a good social worker can help.

Resources

Cook Books and Articles

A Taste of the Good Life: A Cookbook for an Interstitial Cystitis Diet, Beverly Laumann (Refer to Laumann's column "Fresh Tastes" featured on the IC Network website.)

Confident Choices: A Cookbook for IC and OAB, Julie Beyer, M.A., R.D.

Confident Choices: Customizing the Interstitial Cystitis Diet, Julie Beyer, M.A., R.D.

The Happy Bladder Cookbook: Cooking for Interstitial Cystitis, Mia Elliot

Fit N Fresh, Mia Elliot

The Happy Bladder Christmas Cookbook, Mia Elliot

The ICN's IC Chef Cookbook

(Blog) *Simply Delicious: Low-Acid Eating Made Simple,* www.icdietproject.com

"The Fibromyalgia Diet: Eating for a Better Quality of Life," article in *ProHealth* online magazine, March 13, 2002, Colleen Black-Brown • www.prohealth.com

(You can order books from the IC Network or Amazon.com.)

Products

Dr. Ching-Yao Shi's Chinese Herbal Tea
(800) 558-9833 • www.acupuncturephilly.com

Pyramid Herb Seasoning/Mediterranean Salad
(Available at Walmart)

Chapter Three

RECLAIMING COMFORT IN YOUR BODY

When the body loses its natural resilience and strength from an ongoing inflammatory process such as IC/BPS, everyday activities can become a challenge. Even sitting in any one position or on an uneven or hard surface for too long can increase tension and pain.

Sitting and IC/BPS

When you sit, your pelvis and low back become the natural base of support for your upper body. But, when pelvic and lower back muscles are weakened by an inflammatory process in the bladder, the abdominal and hip flexor (front of the hips) muscles must work harder to provide postural support. For example, many IC/BPS patients find that they must sit with their hips rolled slightly back and under to ease the pressure on the pelvic floor and bladder. However, this rather collapsed position forces a head forward posture and the abdominal and hip flexor muscles end up tensing to hold the posture. In time these muscles will shorten and become thick and weak (contributing to the IC/BPS belly) as they work harder to maintain a comfortable sitting position. When you add upper body movements, such as typing and desk work, this postural compensation increases. Using a supportive chair, a comfortable seat cushion that provides support for both the lower and upper back, as well as a foot rest to elevate your feet, can take pressure off of your pelvic floor and bladder, and allow your abdominal muscles to go into slack and relax, which will prevent muscle shortening.

The IC Network sells seat cushions for IC/BPS patients. The company Current Medical Technologies (www.cmtme.com) carries a cushion called the Thera-Seat, which is also recommended for IC/BPS patients. These cushions are helpful to patients with prostatitis and pudendal nerve inflammation.

Table and desk heights should always be considered as well. IC/BPS patients often need to cross their legs for extra support while sitting. Although this practice is not encouraged by doctors and therapists, patients should allow enough room under desks and tables to accommodate crossed, stretched out, and elevated legs.

Sitting for periods of time is hard on the lumbar spine (low back), the pelvic floor muscles, and hip flexors, so standing and practicing intermittent stretching every twenty to thirty minutes is necessary to avoid stiffness. But, before standing it's important to release the accumulated tension in the small muscles of the neck and shoulders. To do so:

Neck and Shoulder Release

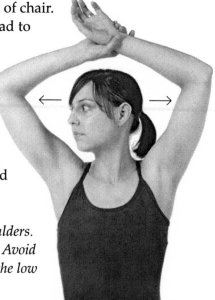

- Push buttocks to the back of chair.
- Lift arms directly over head to un-weight shoulders and relax lower back.
- Grasp and secure one wrist, then rotate head side to side.
- Lead the rotation with eyes. After several rotations grasp other wrist and repeat.

Avoid moving arms and shoulders. Move only the neck and head. Avoid lifting shoulders and arching the low back. This exercise can be done sitting or standing anytime you feel tension in your neck and shoulders.

Support for Standing and Walking

When you are standing, your feet become your base of support. If your abdominal, hip flexor, and hamstring muscles (the large muscles in the back of your legs) are short, tight, and weak, your body's weight will have a tendency to fall back into the heels. In this posture, walking can cause a jarring impact to your pelvic floor, and forward movement, such as walking and climbing stairs, becomes dependent on already tightened hip flexors.

Because these muscular restrictions affect posture, it's very important to pay attention to the style of shoes you wear. Shoes affect your knees and hips and shape your upper body posture. Wearing the right shoes assists forward movement and reduces the impact on your pelvic floor when you are standing and walking. Ideally, IC/BPS patients should wear lightweight shoes with rubber soles that have a little lift in the heels. Patients should avoid shoes and sandals that have negative heels (heels lower than toes). Negative heels place the body's weight back into the heels which increases the impact of walking. Thong sandals, as well as sandals and shoes with high-cut insteps, also place body weight back in the heels. Shoes must feel comfortable when first trying on and walking around the store. Patients should never buy shoes that need "breaking in."

For optimum support, always match your shoes to your tasks. For example, driving moccasins are comfortable for driving but they won't provide support while walking. Be mindful and reevaluate your shoes periodically. Unwelcomed shifts in body distribution can occur with pregnancy, perimenopause, age, weight gain, injury, and medical conditions, such as IC/BPS and fibromyalgia (FMS). If you spend most of your time at home, wear supportive slippers or comfortable supportive shoes. You can always place foam insoles in shoes and slippers for more cushioning.

Comfort and Support While Lying Down

Your whole body is supported when you are lying down. Unfortunately, night can be the most uncomfortable time for patients with urinary frequency. It's not only tiring getting in and out of bed to use the bathroom, it's difficult to let your body relax when you have a constant awareness of your bladder and the surrounding muscles. Sleeping on a mattress that's not too hard can help muscles to rest comfortably and "let go." But, soft or uneven mattresses will make matters worse because they cause muscles to tense as they try to find support for relaxation.

Mattresses with cotton tops or individually pocketed coils can reduce movement and encourage deep sleep. Memory-foam mattresses are questionable because the foam contours to your posture, which may be compromised by musculature restriction. Sleeping with a pillow between your knees can help reduce hip pain if you are a side sleeper. However, it's best to use a baby pillow instead of a standard size which can put pressure on your hips. Using the Aston concept of placing a flat baby pillow between your waist and arm pit can reduce both hip and shoulder pain when lying on your side. Hugging any size pillow when sleeping on your side can reduce shoulder and neck pain. Sleeping is repair time. Make your mattress and pillows a priority so you can get as much quality sleep as possible. *Refer to Chapter Six to avoid mattresses containing toxic materials.*

Body Mechanics for IC/BPS

Begin each day by warming your spinal muscles and discs. This morning ritual will help minimize stiffness upon rising:

Morning Rotations
- Sit on the side of the bed. Place feet comfortably apart on the floor, or bed frame if feet don't reach the ground. Bend elbows and touch finger tips. Imagine arms resting on a shelf.
- Relax shoulders and gently rotate upper body side to side. Lead the movement with eyes so that head turns first.

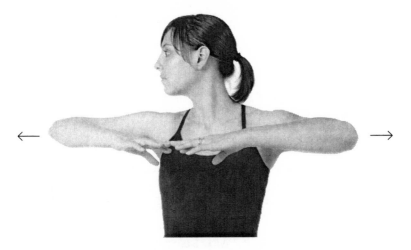

- Begin with four rotations a day and then work up to a comfortable number of repetitions.

Avoid arching low back and lifting shoulders.

Since the bladder is the most active in the morning and early hours of the afternoon, IC/BPS patients should be cautious not to physically overextend or practice challenging exercise during this time. Patients with fibromyalgia (FMS) also wake up with stiffness as well as fibro fog. Stressing stiff and weak muscles can lead to uneven tone and the inability for muscles to find a normal resting position after use. Patients should learn to use their legs for proper support while bending and lifting to avoid overstretching their muscles. If the low back and hips are especially tight and weak, bringing the knees together before bending forward or lifting provides extra support and stability. Ideally, IC/BPS patients should strengthen their leg and gluteal (buttocks) muscles to help with everyday activities.

Patients should also be mindful of their tasks and arrange desks and tabletops to suit their needs. Twisting and reaching should be avoided. So should leaning and lifting one hip off of a chair. Work and chairs need to be lined up. Headsets or speaker phones can be used to prevent stressing the shoulders, neck, and arms.

Patients with "whole body" IC/BPS and/or FMS may want to use a laptop computer instead of a computer with a mouse. A laptop allows equal use of the arms and hands, resulting in less uneven repetition and tension. Of course, a lower chair may be needed or the laptop may have to be raised or adjusted to prevent neck strain and a collapsed posture.

When core strength (abdominal, back, and buttock muscles) is compromised, objects should be carried close to the body with both arms and shouldn't be very heavy, otherwise lifting may aggravate the bladder, the hips, stress the neck, shoulder, and arm joints, and/or result in tiny tears in muscle cells, which is a real concern for patients with FMS. Learning to problem solve, using proper body support and mechanics, keeping physical goals realistic, and maintaining strength will help to reduce the overall effects of IC/BPS and overlapping conditions.

Patients should avoid exercising within two hours of their bedtime. Exercise elevates the body's temperature, which can interfere with sleep.

Exercise and IC/BPS

The right type of exercise is a beneficial ingredient in pain management. Exercise promotes mood-enhancing hormones, such as endorphins, the natural opiates that help to block the perception of pain. Aerobic activity has been found to jog the brain's endocannabinoid system, another mood-enhancing system. There are also many other perks of exercise, including improved strength and balance, deeper breathing and better circulation, a better quality of sleep, easier digestion and elimination, and a better chance of fighting off infection, all of which reduce both physical and mental stress. However, the wrong type of exercise can lead to uneven tone, pain, inactivity, and sometimes an increase in bladder symptoms. Trying to find a realistic and comfortable form of exercise for IC/BPS can be a bit like playing the child's game "Mother May I," because IC/BPS expresses itself differently in patients. Patients with symptoms mostly localized to their bladders may be more capable of performing strenuous exercise, such as lifting weights while sitting or standing. Other IC/BPS patients with a more systemic syndrome, such as FMS, or patients who experience fatigue, joint and muscle pain, and/or a weak and shaky feeling in their core after physical activity may need to *avoid* forms of exercise that require the following:

- imposed postures and movements (workout machines)
- lifting the knees and/or kicking while sitting or standing
- turning the knees inward toward the center of the body
- eccentric movements (stretching a muscle while also contracting or working it, for example, loading a dishwasher, vacuuming, lifting objects over the head, or holding and moving hand and/or leg weights straight out from body)

Jill Osborne of the IC Network believes that the StairMaster is one of the most challenging workout machines for IC/BPS patients.

Fortunately, patients today have many options for exercise that re-educates and strengthens muscles. Yoga is a very popular form of muscle re-education that restores both strength and flexibility. However, the different forms of yoga should be considered.

According to Susi Buhmann, P.T., FMS patients should steer clear of Astanga, Power, or Hot Yoga. "Any type of yoga that is based on non-stop movements is not tolerated well by FMS patients," says Buhmann. Patients need to follow gentle forms, such as *Restorative* and *Hatha* yoga.

Restorative yoga offers stress-reducing benefits, teaching passive stretching and using supportive props. *Hatha* yoga involves more activity, using both stretching and strengthening. *Hatha* yoga classes range from gentle to vigorous. Before participating in a new beginner's yoga class, patients need to view the class to see how much tension is held in the posture. Some yoga instructors teach their students to hyperextend (arch) their lower backs, lifting their rib cages very high, and pulling their pelves under.

(Many IC/BPS patients already have posterior pelves.) These holding and lifting patterns cause extra tension in the body and are not necessary for yoga postures. A more relaxed and supportive posture in yoga positions will have similar results without the imposed effort. An instructor who has experience with chronic pain patients won't be so idealistic about the abilities of her or his students. If attending a yoga class is too challenging, there are instructors trained in *Yoga therapy* who teach individuals with specific needs.

Pilates is another very popular and widely practiced mind/body exercise. One of the main principals of *Pilates* is the focus on core stability. During abdominal exercise participants are asked to scoop their bellies to their spines. But, when abdominal muscles are held in this contraction for sustained periods of time, the pelvic floor (the hammock supporting the pelvic organs), sacrum (the triangular bone at the bottom of the spine), piriformis (hip rotator), and coccyx (tailbone) will tighten at the joints. In some instances, *Pilates* may actually shorten core muscles and IC/BPS patients already have shortened core muscles.

Recognizing this problem, IC/BPS patient, Jennifer Lelwica Buttaccio, O.T.R./L., created *New Dawn Pilates for People with Pelvic Pain.* Buttaccio's DVD offers short sections which allow patients to personalize their workout according to their capabilities. With thorough instruction, she shows patients how to use support for their movements. Buttaccio also demonstrates stretching and tension releasing exercises intermittently throughout each segment. *New Dawn Pilates* benefits patients who experience symptoms localized to the pelvic area. *To order* New Dawn Pilates *see Resources.*

Aston Pilates offers a modified version of Pilates based on Aston Principals, such as proper base of support, cooperation of body parts, and optimal alignment and tone. *Aston Pilates* uses the natural asymmetry of the body instead of imposing rigid postures and movements. Instructors teach students how to unwind their individual tension patterns (so they don't build muscle in a tension pattern) while gently strengthening and lengthening their core muscles. *See Resources.*

Muscle re-education is a process and should begin thoughtfully and slowly. To experience a gentle movement routine, which combines Yoga, Pilates, and Aston-Patterning Principals, refer to the following exercise routine. When practiced as a flowing movement ritual, the exercises stretch, strengthen, and release core and pelvic floor muscles using the most beneficial forms of support. While learning the exercises, only hold the stretches for a breath or two. Begin strengthening movements with only four repetitions (on each side if applies). As you become familiar with the routine, you can hold the stretches for a longer count and slowly increase the number of strengthening repetitions. In order to prevent stiffness and injury, it's necessary to warm your muscles before stretching and strengthening, and never force or repeat a movement that causes discomfort or pain.

Gentle Stretching and Strengthening for Core and Pelvic Floor Muscles

Illustration of towel

FLAT TOWEL

→

→

Before beginning, fold a standard bath size towel in half. Then fold it in half again. When you are ready to use the towel, place it under your hips, about a couple of inches *above* the waistline, which will help to relax your lower back. When using the towel while you are on all fours, roll the towel ends and curl your fingers around the ends to avoid jamming your elbows and shoulders.

Easy Warm-Up

Take a brisk walk around your house or apartment. Feel movement in your whole body (including your head) as you walk. Swing your arms from your elbows and not from your shoulders. Take a few air punches. Avoid making sharp turns.

1) Full Body Stretch

Lie on your back *without* the folded towel. Bend one knee and extend the other leg and the arm opposite the extended leg. Inhale, exhale, and feel your back sink into the floor. Next, rock your extended leg in and out leading the movement with your foot. Repeat on other side.

*Avoid straightening your extended arm. Relax your shoulder. Avoid leading the rocking with your knee. Rock your thigh instead.

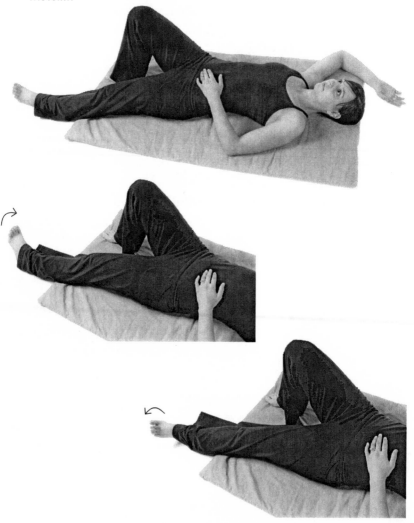

2) Hamstring Stretch

Place the folded towel under buttocks about 1½ to two inches above the waistline.

Bend both knees with feet on the floor "hip width apart." Lift one leg over the hip and lace hands below the knee on the back of the thigh. Inhale, exhale, and push heel to ceiling and curl toes toward face. Repeat with other leg.

**Avoid tucking chin,
tensing elbows and shoulders.*

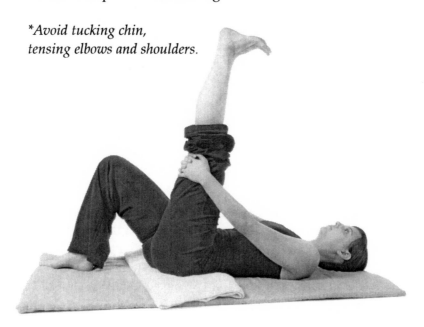

3) Hip Stretch

Bend both knees with feet "hip width apart." Cross one leg in front of the other. Place hand around your ankle (or close to it), and the other hand against the knee. Keeping calf parallel to floor, slowly inhale, exhale, and push knee away from body. Keep ankle stabilized with other hand. Allow head to roll to most comfortable side. Repeat with other leg.

**Avoid tensing shoulders and elbows or holding stretch more
than 15 counts. Place a folded towel or flat pillow under head if
needed to help shoulders and elbows relax.*

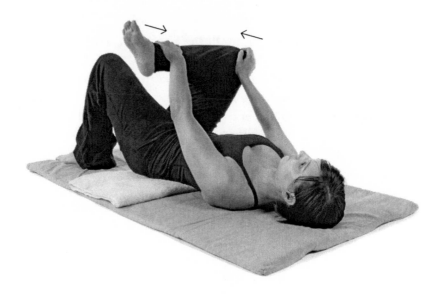

4) Knee Hug Rock

Bring knees to chest and hug them. Gently rock side to side, leading the movement with your eyes so your head turns first. Feel the movement massage your back.

Avoid rocking too slowly. The movement should flow back and forth.

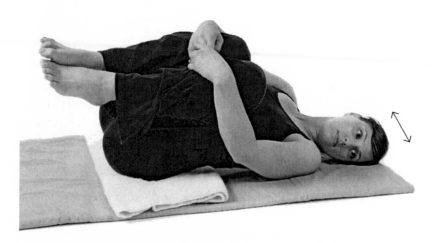

5) Leg Pumps

Place hands under buttocks on towel and bring knees toward chest. Pump legs in and out. Let your head slightly roll to the side when bringing knees toward chest so you don't tighten your neck.

*Avoid tucking chin and extending legs out at a low angle (which will stress the abdominals).

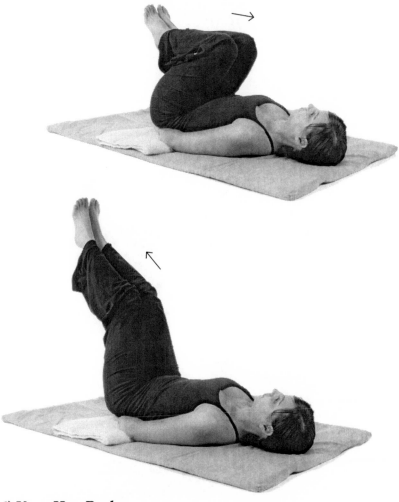

6) Knee Hug Rock

Repeat #4.

7) Bicycle

Bring knees into chest. Place finger tips on the sides of your head. Gently bicycle legs in the air, turning head and elbow toward opposite knee as it cycles in toward body.

> *Avoid extending legs at a low angle and lifting your head, which may put too much strain on your lower abdomen and bladder. Build repetitions very slowly. (If you feel shaky and weak in your abdomen after performing this exercise, discontinue it, but continue practicing the rest of the routine. You may be able to add it back in later when your body becomes stronger.)*

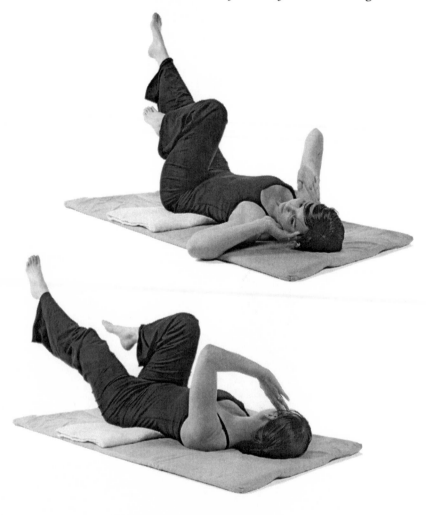

8) Knee Hug Rock

Repeat #4.

9) Happy Baby

After Knee Hug Rock, lift feet into the air with knees bent. Grab hold of your big toes or balls of feet. Hold for a few breaths.

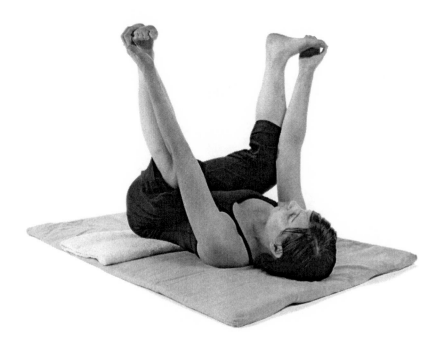

10) Lotus Rock

Bend knees out to sides and loosely hold ankles (or close to ankles). Rest bent arms on thighs and gently rock side to side. Lead rock with eyes, so head turns first. Gently push thighs out with arms while rocking. When finished, rock body over to one side and push yourself up onto all fours.

*Avoid tensing shoulders

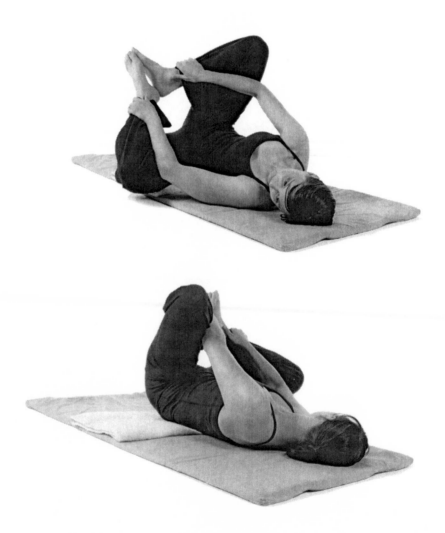

11) Stretch and Crawl

On all fours, rest buttocks down toward or onto bent legs. Keep head and neck relaxed and aligned with spine. Stretch arms out in front of body on floor. (You will not need a towel for this stretch.) Lift buttocks off legs by crawling forward with fingers. Hold position while resisting with fingers, then allow hips to pull body slowly back onto legs while still using resistance.

*Avoid forcing buttocks down onto legs.

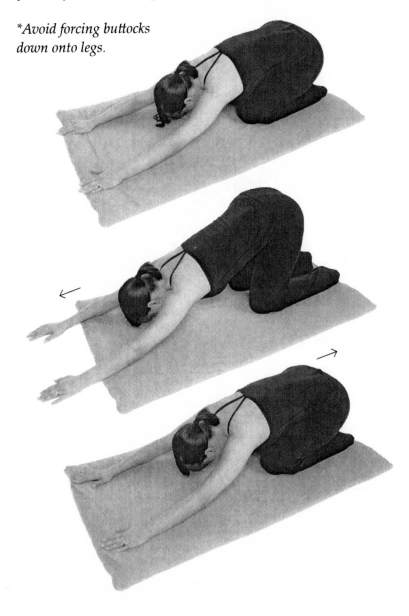

12) Opposite Arm and Leg Extension

With legs hip width apart and hands curled around the edges of the towel, lift opposite arm and leg. Do not straighten extended arm. Keep it slightly bent with hand facing inward. Relax shoulders and head. Focus eyes on outstretched hand. Repeat on other side. Work up to holding the position for a count of ten, or use active alternating repetitions of the position.

*Avoid lifting or dropping head or locking elbows. Keep neck and back aligned. Do not lift leg higher than the spine.

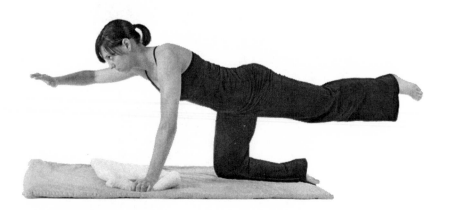

13) Glute Kicks

Bend one knee and bring nose back toward knee. Spring body forward while kicking leg straight back. Repeat movement and then repeat with the other leg.

*Avoid lifting head. Keep back and neck aligned. Avoid locking elbows.

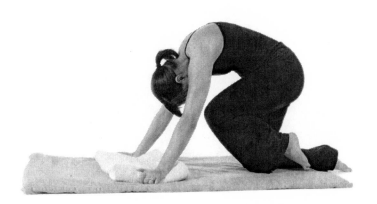

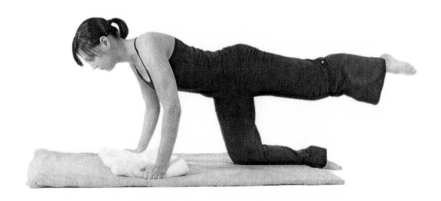

14) Rest Pose

Back on all fours, with legs hip width apart, flex upper body and rest back on legs. Bend elbows and place one hand on top of the other. Rest forehead on hands. Hold position.

Avoid tensing shoulders or forcing buttocks down. Flex feet if cramping occurs.

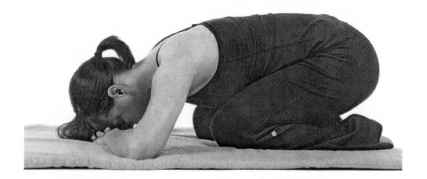

15) Glute Lifts

With neck aligned with spine, bend one leg with foot flexed toward ceiling. Shift slightly forward while lifting the bent knee toward the ceiling. Bring knee back down to starting position and repeat.

*Avoid locking elbows. Intermittenly straighten and shake out legs if hamstring muscles cramp.

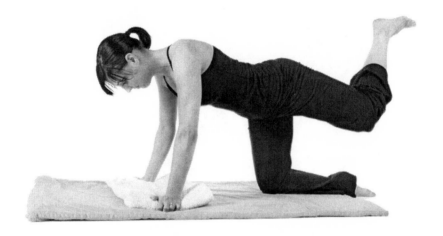

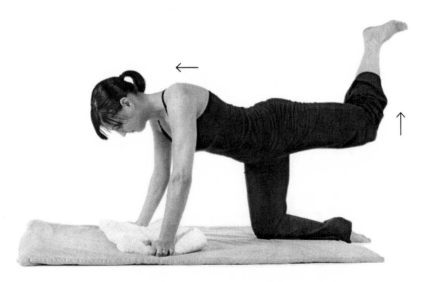

16) Hip Stretch

Cross one leg in front of the other, then rest down on elbows. Slide back leg straight behind. Upper body follows down to floor. Hold only long enough to get into position. Push up with hands, take a deep breath and change legs.

*Avoid forcing hips down toward floor. Keep neck relaxed. Avoid this exercise if you have knee problems.

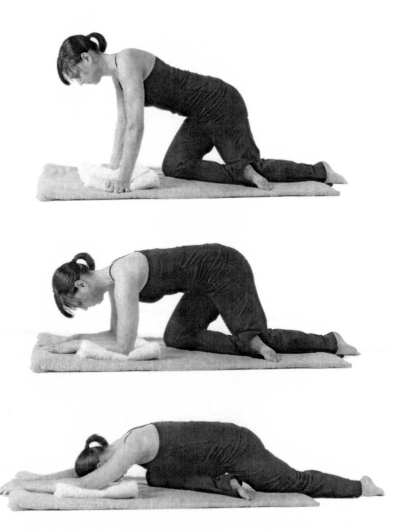

17) Drinking Lion

Keep knees "hip width" apart. Face hands inward. Swoop upper body forward and down with face close to hands. Hold position.

Avoid holding tension in neck.

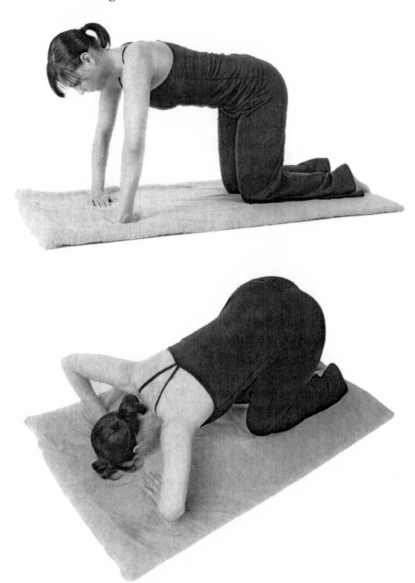

18) Downward Facing Dog

Push your body up so hands and feet are on the floor. Slightly bend elbows. Relax head and neck. Hold position.

*Avoid tensing elbows and forcing heels to floor. Avoid locking knees.

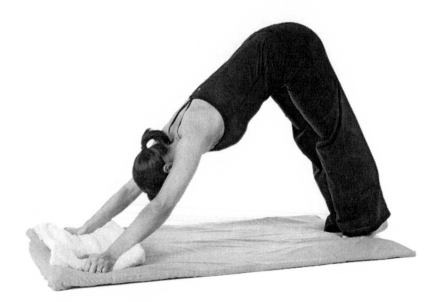

19) Hip Stretch Kneeling

Kneel on one knee. Bend the other leg and place foot on floor slightly in front of the knee above. Tuck pelvis under and shift knee forward over foot. Hold and repeat on other side.

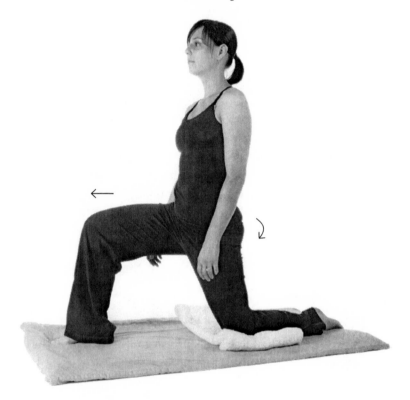

20) Neck and Shoulder Stretch

Begin by standing with arms in front of body. Clasp and secure one wrist with opposite hand. Gently pull down on secured wrist and tilt head toward the shoulder opposite the held wrist (ear toward shoulder). Keep chin centered. Hold position. Repeat stretch with other arm. Then follow the same stretches with arms behind back (which is shown here).

Avoid lifting chin or shoulders, arching low back, and locking knees. When learning this stretch, practice in front of a mirror to get head centered.

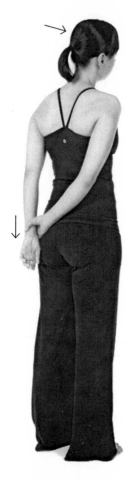

After practicing this routine take another brisk walk around your home and notice easier movement and a lighter feeling in your body. If needed, use an ice pack on stiff or sore muscles after exercise.

It is *essential* for IC/BPS patients to continually encourage range of motion, flexion and extension of the spine, and length and strength in the muscles. Moderate aerobic activity, such as walking, swimming, water exercise, or dancing to dance videos, is also necessary for optimum relief and strength. However, walking can be a challenge when pelvic floor and hip flexor muscles are tight and hips are imbalanced and misaligned. Maintaining a suitable stretching and strengthening routine can help to loosen muscles, align hips, and make walking easier. Soft tissue work and trigger point therapy can also help to make movement easier.

Swimming is a great aerobic activity because the whole body is supported. Aquatic exercise programs are usually gentle enough for chronic pain patients. As always, patients should start at beginner's level and view classes before signing up. Dancing on the right surface (not a concrete floor) to realistic types of music, such as "the oldies" is very energizing and a fun form of aerobic exercise.

Whatever form of exercise patients choose, they should practice that form regularly, at least three to four times a week. *See Resources for information on Pilates, aquatic programs, and an instructive walking DVD.*

Some patients cannot tolerate pools that are disinfected with chlorine and need to find pools that use alternative disinfectants, such as salt. Patients participating in aquatic classes may need to stand in water that covers their shoulders when performing arm exercises.

Resources

Videos and Programs

New Dawn Pilates, Volume 1: A Pilates-Inspired Workout Adapted for People with Pelvic Pain, Jennifer Buttaccio and Tom Buttaccio (This DVD is available through the IC Network or Amazon.com.)

Aston Pilates Program and *Aston's Walking the New Body* (Video) www.astonkinetics.com • (775) 831-8228

The United States Water Fitness Association (Aquatic programs) www.uswfa.com • (561) 732-9908

Chapter Four

TRYING HANDS-ON, TRADITIONAL, AND ALTERNATIVE THERAPIES

Many female IC/BPS patients initially seek help from their gynecologists, due to confusion about the source of their pain and/or the fact that their gynecologists usually treat their bladder infections. Their gynecologists, in turn, ideally refer these patients to urologists or urogynecologists for relief of their symptoms if they suspect IC/BPS. Although it may take a good bit of time for both female and male patients to find the right doctors, when they finally receive their diagnoses, the first interventions are typically empirical treatments and medications which have been shown to relieve the symptoms of IC/BPS. While these medications and treatments have improved symptoms and life quality for many patients, traditional health-care approaches may not always alleviate patients' symptoms, and there are IC/BPS patients who choose not to limit their treatment to traditional methods. Either way, many of these patients subsequently seek help and pain management from an array of alternative health-care professionals, other than urologists, in their search to relieve and control their symptoms and any accompanying conditions of the illness.

Many doctors who treat newly researched illnesses are grateful to have more to offer their patients. These physicians are most likely to be receptive to complimentary and alternative treatments (CAM) and often feel that IC/BPS is more than just a bladder disease. They also believe that there are therapies besides bladder instillations and medications which have the ability to address the bladder and the whole person.

According to Jill Osborne, IC/BPS patient and president of the IC Network, the patients who have the most success use a combination of traditional and alternative treatments for the symptoms of IC/BPS. This combination is referred to as integrative medicine, which blends evidence-based alternative therapies with traditional medicine.

Alternative health-care approaches are often helpful for treatment of the overlapping conditions of IC/BPS, but like some traditional treatments, they don't always alleviate bladder symptoms. No one treatment, whether alternative or traditional, works for all IC/BPS patients. Genetics, pre-existing injuries and illnesses, personal lifestyles, beliefs, and the treatment or lack of treatment from health-care providers can affect the success of any IC/BPS intervention. The receptiveness of patients to new treatments is often related to the severity of their bladder symptoms. Patients with less sensitive bladders may be more willing to explore a variety of therapies. In contrast, patients with more sensitive bladders face the possibility that new treatments will fail and actually aggravate symptoms. These patients will naturally be more hesitant to try new interventions after having had one-too-many bad experiences.

Even though awareness has vastly improved, there are still health-care practitioners who do not understand IC/BPS and are not flexible enough to listen closely to the unique needs of their IC/BPS patients. This lack of understanding can leave patients feeling alone when they seek help away from the urology or urogynecology office. In addition, there are far too many health-care practitioners who in turn blame IC/BPS patients when there is no improvement from therapy. Not too long ago, some alternative practitioners were trained to believe that the patient was 90 percent responsible for the outcome of the therapy and the practitioner responsible for only 10 percent! Good therapists or health-care practitioners will never promise that they can cure you and will accept the fact that you have a physical illness that is very difficult to treat. In particular, any new age cure-all treatment should be viewed with skepticism because of unrealistic claims.

The roots of alternative medicine lie mostly in ancient Eastern methods of healing and prevention, as well as European behavioral theories and mentalist philosophies handed down from the later nineteenth century and early twentieth century, before the organic nature of many illnesses was recognized. Alternative pioneers carefully broke down many Eastern theories and approaches to health, then reinterpreted and blended these ideas to our Western way of thinking. Beliefs stemming from the behavioral theories of "hysteria" were also broken and blended into a new age of neo-Freudian awareness.

Problems and illnesses in the different organs and parts of the body were considered as psychological in nature and "stress" was recognized as the cause of disease instead of the trigger for disease. For instance, during the 1970s an alternative practitioner may have believed that a nearsighted person's eye difficulties were caused by a trauma during childhood. According to this belief, the trauma would have prevented the eye muscles from developing normally, because the child had withdrawn his or her vision, becoming introverted or too shy to want to see. Misunderstood illnesses affecting women were also labeled as stress disorders. Endometriosis was called the "working-woman's disease" and believed to occur in "type A" personalities (overachievers). Somatization disorders were considered to be physical disorders caused by emotional conflicts, anxiety, and depression which the patient could not confront. Consequently, it was believed that these disorders became unconsciously displaced onto the body, or into the body parts (such as the bladder). Despite this theory, removal of dysfunctional organs was pretty common.

Although stress should not be underestimated in its ability to make us susceptible to illness, it was misunderstood and misconstrued as it worked its way into the psycho-babble of the 1970s. The blaming of the 70s was not limited to the field of alternative medicine. During this time medical students were still being taught that IC/BPS and many other conditions mostly affecting women were of a psychological nature. Treating the mind was extremely popular. While the holistic, or mind/body field, embraced many wonderful treatments and techniques to heal the whole body, Western medical doctors were experimenting with new philosophies and new drugs to treat the mind. This may explain why the alternative field first used the term "body/mind" before it was changed to "mind/body."

Today mind/body medicine has become more sophisticated. Alternative practitioners and teachers have aged and lost some of their idealistic views. Traditional doctors have become more open-minded to chronic pain conditions. Diseases and diagnoses are now better understood by both fields, and harmful beliefs have come a long way from the days when multiple sclerosis was called "faker's disease." As East really meets West, some very wonderful and important techniques from both fields of medicine are being utilized for their powerful benefits. Many different therapies are available to help patients recognize, reduce, and manage the ongoing stress of chronic illness. However, chronic pain patients must be realistic about the therapies they choose and realize that the therapist should be considered as important as the therapy itself. The following information is intended to offer insight into various modalities and how they may or may not be beneficial to IC/BPS patients.

Pelvic Floor Therapy

First considered an alternative treatment, hands-on pelvic floor therapy is now recognized by the traditional medical field as an effective nerve-modulating treatment for pelvic floor dysfunction (PFD) and IC/BPS. PFD is a condition that causes the pelvic floor muscles (which form a hammock that supports and raises the pelvic organs) to involuntarily spasm, making urination, elimination, and sex painful and/or difficult. There are doctors who believe that PFD can be caused by IC/BPS and others who believe that PFD causes IC/BPS. Both could be true since the majority of patients have PFD and the pelvic floor muscles have a close nerve connection to the bladder. (Around two-thirds of all patients with chronic pelvic pain have PFD.)

PFD is diagnosed with a pelvic exam. During the exam (vaginal for women and rectal for men) a doctor or physical therapist can identify areas of point tenderness and tightness, as well as myofascial trigger points that may be causing abnormal contractions of the pelvic floor. (The exam must be done very gently or it can trigger symptoms in the bladder, and referred pain in the hips, low back, and legs.) Trigger points present as nodules, which are contracted knots, and/or or tight bands. They are found in major pelvic floor muscles: the puborectalis, the iliococygeus and pubococcygeus, and the obturator internus, as well as other areas. But, no matter where trigger points or areas of point tenderness are located, the pelvic floor reacts singularly to pain.

> *Trigger points in the iliococygeus and the pubococcygeus can refer the familiar hip pain that so many IC/BPS patients complain about. Physical therapists trained in pelvic floor therapy know to treat these trigger points gently, otherwise severe hip pain can result and become chronic.*

Trigger points can be caused by many things: surgeries, child birth, joint problems, viral infections, injuries such as repetitive motion trauma, and the cold. They can also result from frequent urination as well as cause frequent urination, leading to a vicious cycle of pelvic floor tension. There are two types of trigger points: active and latent. Active trigger points may be sensitive to palpation, but the pain is felt at a distal site. This is called referred pain. Active trigger points can hurt when the muscle involved (a pelvic floor muscle in this case) is used, and very active trigger points can hurt when the muscle is at rest. On the other hand, latent trigger points only hurt when they are pressed, but still can contribute to muscle shortening and weakness, and cause restricted movement. Latent trigger points can also become active when the involved muscles are overstretched or overused (for example, fighting urgency, experiencing frequency, and participating in sexual intercourse).

Active trigger points appear to be responsible for the neurogenic inflammation of the bladder wall and are at the root of pelvic floor tension. When pelvic floor muscles sense pain, such as pain caused by an active trigger point after urination, the bladder nerves become activated and the nerve endings release the excitatory neurotransmitter substance P and other neurotransmitters, which cause mast cell degranulation; mast cells release irritating histamine, serotonin, and prostaglandins, which cause IC/BPS symptoms.

Trigger points should be addressed quickly to prevent widespread pain. Treatment to calm trigger points may include direct and indirect myofascial release, strain/counter strain release (this treatment may not be suitable for all patients), strumming and muscle energy techniques, joint mobilizations, organ-specific fascial mobility (visceral mobilization to improve the functioning of the organs), integrative manual therapy, CranioSacral therapy, strengthening, indirect and direct stretching, neuromuscular re-education, as well as home exercise (tight, weak muscles are more prone to trigger points), self-massage techniques, and relaxation and bladder management. Injections of lidocaine, anti-inflammatory agents, and muscle relaxants can also be used to treat trigger points in the pelvic floor and other areas—as can "dry needling" (without medication) which also helps to release tension.

Patients must keep in mind that many noxious chemicals are released into the bloodstream when trigger points are deactivated. Because of this release, patients must drink plenty of water after any session that addresses trigger points.

Lidocaine has occasionally triggered bladder symptoms in IC/ BPS patients. Some patients may also be sensitive to anti-inflammatory medications, as well as some muscle relaxants that are sometimes injected into trigger points.

Pelvic floor therapy should only be used when patients are ready. (Some therapists prefer to use a numbing agent like topical lidocaine before internal work.) Patients who cannot tolerate internal therapy often get relief from soft tissue release along the lateral edge of the pubic and inferior ramus, the gluteal attachments, the deep lateral rotator muscles (especially the piriformis), and the soft tissue around the ischial tuberosities (sitz bones). However, working too close to the urethra can irritate the pudendal nerve. The pudendal nerve innervates all pelvic floor structures and when it gets irritated or damaged, it can cause pudendal neuralgia and symptoms similar to IC/BPS. Manual techniques, such as "nerve tissue tension releases," and medications for IC/BPS (including some other medications) are often used to relieve pudendal nerve pain. *Refer to Chapter One.*

Physical therapy for IC/BPS patients isn't limited to the pelvic floor. The muscles of the pelvis are made of both the pelvic floor and hip-joint muscles, and have other attachments. Muscular tension, referred pain, and restriction, caused by IC/BPS and pelvic floor dysfunction, can occur in the:

- adductors (inner thighs)
- gluteus (buttocks)
- piriformus (hip rotator and support muscle of the pelvic floor)
- hamstrings (backs of thighs)
- quadriceps (front of thighs)
- iliopsoas (major hip flexor connected to the ribs)
- quadratus (lower back)
- rectus abdominus, external obliques, and the other abdominal muscles

A tight piriformis, which is an important hip rotator, can affect the pudendal nerve. Trigger points in the obliques transversus (abdominal muscles) can be responsible for pain in the pelvis, groin, and perineal area. Trigger points in the rectus abdominus may cause pelvic pain and an increase of intraabdominal pressure. Abdominal muscles assist urination and defecation.

Tight areas and trigger points in these muscles can trigger bladder and pelvic floor symptoms, leading to a vicious cycle. It's obvious that the pelvic floor, hip-joint, leg, lower back, and abdominal muscles be addressed. But, usually when the bladder calms down so do most of the other trigger points.

Ideally, the whole body should be addressed because IC/BPS can cause postural restrictions and compensations. For example, our hips act as the steering wheel for our knees. But, if our hips are restricted by IC/BPS, pelvic floor dysfunction and/or sacroiliac joint dysfunction, our legs and feet, as well as our upper bodies, are affected. Restrictions around the sacral area (where nerves to the bladder are located), and restrictions in the pubic symphysis (where the pubic bones join over the bladder) also contribute to pain and postural problems. A good physical therapist will access and address compensations and rotations in the whole body.

A knowledgeable urologist or urogynecologist can refer IC/BPS patients to physical therapists with training in pelvic floor therapy, or patients can contact the American Physical Therapy Association, the International Organization of Physiotherapists, or the International Pelvic Pain Society for therapists trained in current treatment for IC/BPS.

It's crucial that patients see therapists who have experience with IC/BPS patients. These therapists realize that most IC/BPS patients have a problem with vaginal or anal probes used in electrical stimulation (e-stim), and that all patients must avoid Kegel exercises. Squeezing, holding, and releasing pelvic floor muscles can cause a flare-up of symptoms. However, electrical stimulation modalities, such as cold laser light therapy applied to the external pelvic area, and therapeutic ultrasound applied externally to the pelvic floor, hips, sacral, and lower abdominal area over the bladder can be very effective treatments. The focus of therapy must be aimed at relaxing the muscles and not strengthening them, because the pelvic muscles of patients with IC/BPS and pelvic floor dysfunction are already hypertonus (overly toned and extremely tense). *See Resources.*

> *Some patients may at first feel some discomfort after pelvic floor therapy, but usually this discomfort goes away and then they begin to experience relief.*

Traditional Physical Therapy

Physical therapy (PT) is often prescribed to IC/BPS patients with persistent muscle problems, injuries, or a diagnosis of FMS. PT is especially helpful to IC/BPS patients who cannot exercise due to limited range of motion, muscle, and joint pain. Many IC/BPS patients find they can exercise more comfortably when they receive manual therapy to release the psoas muscle because this large hip flexor connects the lower body to the upper body, running from the inside of the hip to the lower ribs.

A good prescription for PT will include soft tissue mobilization, the myo-therapy most accepted in the medical field. This manipulation focuses on the release of the soft tissues (the fascia which is the connective tissue surrounding the muscles) and can be used on any restricted area.

Well trained physical therapists will use firm, smooth, and blending strokes to encourage trigger point release and even tone. Helping patients to become aware of their own tension patterns and how IC/BPS and/or FMS contribute to these patterns is also very important. Proper loosening, stretching, and possibly e-stim (on the injured or restricted area) must be introduced before gentle strengthening. Sports medicine should almost always be avoided, especially for patients with FMS and those who experience the full body effects of IC/BPS. These patients do not need more physical challenges.

Instead, patients need encouragement, which requires therapists to be more open to the specific limitations of IC/BPS and FMS. These limitations may include the inability to support small hand weights while sitting or standing. (Patients can usually support small weights while lying down.) Experienced therapists will have the ability to modify strength-building exercises and understand that IC/BPS patients with FMS may need different treatment than FMS patients without IC/BPS. Techniques used for FMS, such as "spray and stretch" (used to help muscles loosen, prevent pain while stretching, and regain range of motion by the use of a cold spray), and "trigger point injections" (injections of an anesthetic into tender-point trigger points usually given by a doctor or nurse), may not be helpful to IC/BPS patients. Patients who suffer with the overlapping condition of chemical sensitivity may have a reaction to the spray used in the "spray and stretch" treatment, and some IC/BPS patients may experience bladder symptoms after trigger point injections (such as lidocaine injections). This is not to dismiss the benefits of muscle pain relief. If general muscle pain is much more persistent than bladder pain, then treating the muscle pain may be more beneficial.

> *Before any injection, patients need to ask if the injection contains epinephrine. Epinephrine is a known bladder irritant and is sometimes used to prolong the life of the injected medication.*

Massage

The goal of massage is to increase circulation, reintroduce a feeling of well-being, and recreate a sense of relaxation and comfort that may be lost in the pain cycle of IC/BPS. Experienced massage therapists will be able to facilitate these improvements by loosening tight muscles, encouraging flexibility, and a cooperation of body parts.

Therapists should also take a history of your symptoms, check with you often about the comfort of your position, and the amount of pressure and strokes used during the massage session. Like too many repetitive movements performed during exercise, too many repetitive strokes to one area of the body during a massage session can cause additional tension in a patient with chronic pain. Massage strokes should be firm (not hard) and smooth. The room temperature should be comfortable. A good rule of thumb to follow when working with a therapist is that *if it feels wrong, then it is wrong for you!* Doctors, physical therapists, chiropractors, and reputable massage schools can usually recommend good licensed massage therapists. Be sure to ask for someone who has experience with chronic pain patients.

Myofascial Therapies

Many different myofascial techniques are available to choose from. Although physical therapists typically use soft tissue mobilization, students of physical therapy study various techniques today. Some therapists combine techniques and others are very disciplined in one modality or theory.

So called "bodywork" is not new. It was well developed during the last quarter of the twentieth century. One popular technique used by a number of IC/BPS patients is Myofascial Release, which focuses on releasing the fascia, the supportive connective tissue surrounding the muscles. Another manual therapy that has proven to work well for both fibromyalgia (FMS) and IC/BPS patients is Aston-Patterning. This multifaceted, hands-on work addresses restrictions in soft tissue (fascia, muscles, and tendons), as well as restrictions around and through the joint tissues. Movement education as well as ergonomic and environmental modification are emphasized as practitioners further unravel clients' individual tension patterns. Aston-Patterning practitioners can also provide excellent gentle exterior pelvic floor work to release restriction and pain. To find practitioners specializing in Myofascial Release contact local physical therapy clinics and massage schools. *To locate practitioners specializing in Aston-Patterning, see Resources.* Although there are a limited number of Aston-Patterning practitioners, you may find physical therapists with some training in Aston-Patterning. Ask the training center when you call.

IC/BPS patients should be mindful and pick muscle therapies that use gentle encouragement to lengthen and unravel tight muscles at the client's or patient's own pace. Patients should be cautious of therapies that attempt to impose an ideal body type (shape or posture), also. Many practitioners use deep tissue work to realign the body to provide more postural support; however, because of the ongoing inflammatory process in the bladder, it is usually not wise to try to realign the pelvis. Practitioners and therapists must be told this before agreeing to a session. Signing up and paying for a series of sessions before experiencing a particular bodywork is not a good idea.

Deep tissue work should mostly be limited to tightened areas around the joints (direct pressure to the joints should be avoided). Surrounding muscles should be blended with firm, smooth strokes. Deep tissue work can help to break up scar tissue or adhesions, and the referred tension of IC/BPS, but may cause too much change for the patient with an inflammatory process in her or his bladder.

When work is too deep or a session is too long, patients may experience spasms and/or exhaustion for a couple of days after, or a new cycle of pain may begin. IC/BPS patients with FMS or the systemic effects of IC/BPS often do not have the tone to support their structural muscles and surrounding tissue after they have been released, so they may end up tensing their already tightened deep muscles and corresponding joints for strength. As a result, patients may end up with a "rag doll" effect. Also, if one specific area of the body is overworked or "overly loosened," other muscles can end up in a tight tension pattern in order to compensate for the imbalance.

IC/BPS patients should avoid therapies that combine hands-on techniques with psychotherapy during the same session. Such techniques are designed to break emotional holding patterns that have settled in the body. Success with psychotherapy is best achieved when clients or patients are free to feel emotions at their own comfortable pace. Emotional patterns usually release naturally with proper myofascial therapy. Most massage or myofascial therapists are not licensed or trained in psychotherapy, therefore this combined technique can be harmful when specific theories are imposed on clients.

For more information about pelvic therapies see "Medical Diagnosis and Treatment" in Chapter Eight.

CranioSacral Treatment

CranioSacral (CSI) therapy is defined as a gentle, hands-on method of evaluating and enhancing the functioning of a physiological body system called the craniosacral system. This system is composed of the membranes (the dura) and cerebrospinal fluid that pulses with a specific rhythm. Both surround and protect the brain and spinal cord. Using very gentle movements, practitioners release restrictions in the craniosacral system (the cranium, the spine, and the sacrum). Releasing these restrictions is intended to calm an upregulated sympathetic nervous system, which is the case with IC/BPS and related conditions.

CSI practitioners may also use visceral manipulation to release abnormal tone and adhesions that work against the organs (the bladder), muscular membranes, and fascia. CSI is occasionally used by doctors and other health-care practitioners, such as physical therapists and osteopaths, and is also combined with other bodywork techniques, like Aston-Patterning. *See Resources.*

Although many IC/BPS patients find they can fully void after a session, patients with systemic IC/BPS, and/or FMS, should caution CSI practitioners to avoid holding their heads too far forward while cradling to feel the pulse of the craniosacral system. Traction should be gentle and as brief as possible.

Osteopathic Manipulative Medicine

Doctors of osteopathic medicine (D.O.) focus on wellness and disease prevention in the whole body much like alternative practitioners, but they can also prescribe drugs and surgery. Osteopaths, who practice manual manipulation, use palpitation and manipulative techniques on the bones, muscles, joints, fascia, and organs to alleviate painful conditions and restore natural function in the body. Osteopathic medicine has been shown to relieve symptoms in some IC/BPS patients.

Chiropractic

Good chiropractic care is another approach to relieving muscular and neurological problems. Gentle adjustments to the lumbar spine (low back), for voluntary bladder function, and the sacrum (the triangular bone at the bottom of the spine), for involuntary bladder function, can help balance overall bladder health. Other vertebrae adjustments often also help. For example, when the lumbar and sacrum cannot be adjusted because of malfunctioning of these joints, a chiropractor may adjust the first vertebrae in the neck and the third thoracic vertebrae (upper back) to aid in balancing the bladder.

An experienced chiropractor will use releasing techniques (massage and/or stretching) to relax tight ligaments and muscles around the adjusted joints, as well as encourage flexion and extension. A full adjustment may have to be broken up into two visits, depending on the tightness of the muscles. Ideally, patients should alternate chiropractic visits with massage sessions. Patients should also practice gentle stretching and toning to keep their spinal alignments.

Chiropractic adjustments sometimes help to break the pain cycle of IC/BPS, because they can release an exaggerated sympathetic nervous system response to a small muscle pull or twist. Sympathetic responses (in which the whole body tenses as it prepares for fight or flight) can affect patients with systemic symptoms, such as FMS.

A well respected New Orleans based chiropractor, Sylvi Beaumont, D.C., has found that men with IC/BPS respond especially well to chiropractic adjustments.

Homeopathy

Homeopathy is a non-drug treatment that uses naturally occurring essences of plant, mineral, or animal origin to treat illness and pain. Homeopathy is based on the concept that "like cures like." This concept is the same idea used in allergy and immunization shots. The homeopath, naturopath, or other health practitioner administers a small dose of a homeopathic remedy to stimulate the body's natural immune defenses and the healing process.

Homeopathy works from the top of the body to the bottom of the body, and from the inside to the outside. Because homeopaths prescribe remedies specifically for the individual, patients who take prescription drugs may benefit from a homeopath who is also an M.D. Homeopaths who are physicians can have a better understanding of the relationship between the patient and the disease, and the role of the patient's prescription medicine. Although homeopathic remedies may be helpful to IC/BPS patients, homeopaths look for specific emotional events, or experiences that correlate with the symptoms and onset of their patients' illnesses rather than simply focusing on healing the physical aspects of the disease. For instance, a homeopath may believe that patients who first suffered with IC/BPS after sexual activity may experience symptoms from sexual guilt.

Chinese Medicine

Acupuncture is a deep energy therapy which is gaining popularity for the treatment of both acute and chronic pain and is known to relieve symptoms in a number of IC/BPS and chronic prostatitis (CP/CPPS) patients. During an acupuncture session, thin needles are placed in specific points of the body to adjust the imbalanced flow of energy called *Qi* (pronunciation: "chee") and also restore the balance that illness has interfered with. Acupuncture helps to release endorphins that fight pain and is thought to help the bladder by regulating the blood supply, which increases beneficial oxygen and nutrients. This increase is important for patients with frequency, because the constant voiding decreases the amount of oxygen and nutrients flowing to the bladder.

A conservative approach to acupuncture is essential for IC/BPS patients because the needles manipulated during a session may be too strong and stimulating for those prone to anxiety. Practitioners should be made aware of this problem and should avoid only beginning with the acupuncture points for the bladder. Practitioners should also be willing to check frequently with their patients who are usually left alone after the needles are placed.

Acupuncture sessions need to be every other day for the first ten sessions. Otherwise, they may be less effective, because the effects can weaken between the sessions. If a patient experiences improvement after the ten-day series, sessions should be continued periodically for maintenance.

To find a licensed or certified acupuncturist, patients should contact a local Acupuncture Association. For the best results an acupuncturist should have at least 500 hours of training as opposed to the 250 hours of training that is routine with many practicing acupuncturists. An Asian practitioner will usually have the most training and understanding of Chinese medicine.

Homeopaths typically believe that acupuncture and other energy therapies should not be initiated at the same time as homeopathy.

Herbal Medicine is usually used by well-trained acupuncturists, as well as other practitioners, to correct an imbalanced body condition and enhance the healing process. In Chinese medicine everything, including the body, is divided into two opposite parts: yin and yang. Yin refers to female and represents dark, passive, cold (water), downward, contracting, and weak energy. Yang implies male and represents bright, strong, hot, upward, active, and expanding energy. A good example of yin and yang is an onion. A cooked onion is yin—watery, and a raw onion is yang—strong, hot (which explains why most IC/BPS patients must avoid raw onions). Illness supposedly occurs when there is an imbalance between yin and yang, as well as other influences in the body.

Treatment is determined by the diagnosis of imbalance in a particular condition inside the body, e.g. urine with a deep yellow color usually indicates an excess-heat condition (inflammation) while clear and profuse urine often reflects an empty-cold condition. Imbalances are revealed by observation of the condition such as the patient's expression, color, appearance, and tongue, by auscultation (listening) and olfaction (smell), by inquiring, and by palpation of the patient's pulse. As with IC/BPS, conditions or imbalances in the body may occur from different causes, but symptoms may be similar in patients. Plants, including roots, barks, seeds, leaves, and flowers that match the imbalance (and/or acupuncture) are prescribed to bring the body back to harmony in order to heal.

Practitioners trained in Chinese medicine believe that mostly women experience imbalances in the urinary systems because of an imbalance between the Liver and the Kidney systems. (Chinese Medicine Theory holds that both the Liver and the Kidney are from the same source and that the Kidney has an external-internal connection with the bladder.) This theory also supports that this imbalance affects the emotions. The abundance of nerves in the bladder area is as well blamed for causing emotional problems when there is an imbalance. According to Chinese medicine, dampness is generally formed by abnormal distribution of body fluids, and the culmination of dampness (yin) could result in a malfunctioning of the bladder system and this malfunction, which may affect the muscles or the lining of the bladder, can occur after an illness such as the flu. (Many IC/BPS patients first experience their IC/BPS symptoms after childbirth, surgery, illness, bladder infection, or a stressful event.)

Tinctures (which contain alcohol), teas, tablets, tonics, and sitz baths have long been used for treatment of bladder disorders in both Eastern and Western medicine. However, finding the proper herb that will work for IC/BPS patients should not be left up to most practitioners as it is still "trial by error" and very individual. Patients with severe pain should understand that only proper herbs can mask bladder pain as effectively as prescription drugs. Patients who are very sensitive to foods and medicines should also know that certain herbs can have an over-relaxing, contracting, burning, or stimulating effect on the bladder. A good practitioner will work with a patient to find the herbal match for the individual's condition. *See Chapter Two and Chapter Six for more information.*

Diet is another aspect of Chinese medicine. Practitioners find that eating the right foods can balance the whole body system. Nerve inflammation and stimulation of the bladder are thought to be corrected with the right foods, along with acupuncture and herbs. Interestingly, some practitioners believe that the nature of food can be changed by the body's digestive juices and urine.

Chinese practitioners, like Chicago-based Wen Xuan, refer to Wu-Wei/Five Properties of food nutrients when balancing the body. These Properties are: spicy, sour, bitter, sweet, and salty. Foods containing these different properties affect the body's functioning. Foods, like herbs, are used to treat the systems that are out of balance. The Five Properties relate to the different systems.

Generally speaking, after foods are digested, the sour nutrient goes to the liver and gallbladder, the bitter nutrient enters the heart and the small intestine, the sweet nutrient reaches the spleen and the stomach, the pungent nutrient goes to the lung and the large intestine, and the salty nutrient moves to the kidney and the bladder. But, when a certain system is imbalanced, the foods that go to that particular system should be avoided. For example:

- The Liver System—foods with the sour property should be avoided
- The Cardio-Vascular System—foods with the bitter property should be removed
- The Digestive System—foods with the sweet property should be removed
- The Respiratory System—foods with the pungent property should be eliminated
- The Urinary, Reproductive, or Endocrine System—foods with the salty property should be avoided

When diseases of the organs are involved, there are general principles of food selection in diet therapy for these diseases:

- Foods with pungent property should be avoided if there is liver disease.
- Foods with salty property should be avoided if there is heart disease.
- Foods with sour property should be avoided if there is spleen disease.
- Foods with sweet properties should be avoided if there is kidney disease.
- Foods with bitter property should be avoided if there is lung disease.

Some of the listed foods to avoid for different diseases are obvious, such as salty foods for heart disease (blood pressure) and sweet foods for kidney disease (diabetes), but what explains the foods that need to be avoided when there is only an imbalance?

A surprising example is the Respiratory System. Although a cold is called a cold, Chinese medicine believes that when a person suffers an imbalance in the Respiratory System, there is heat deep inside of the system, which explains why he or she should avoid pungent foods (hot and spicy). Another example: when the Urinary, Reproductive, or Endocrine System is imbalanced, salty foods should be avoided. Why, because salt retains water in the body. However, the opposite holds true when a person's body is in balance. These properties (in foods) become nourishing to the systems. Refer to the following:

- **SWEET** nourishes the Spleen and Stomach—foods that are considered sweet and are bladder-safe for many patients are: grains, millet (Xiao Mi), rice, squashes, long bean, bean sprouts, white onions (cooked), blueberries, figs (WuHuaGuo), potato, celery, soy bean, honey, pear, carrots, lotus root, lotus seed, mung bean, milk, chicken, pork, oyster, eggs, belt fish, shrimp, octopus, clam, sugar, wine (late harvest sweet wine only), etc.
- **SOUR** nourishes the Liver and Gallbladder—some of the sour foods include: barley (DaMai), turkey, green olives (without vinegar or citric acid), red bean, pear, lotus seed, etc. Vinegar is usually used for sour flavor but as you can see there are other bladder-safe foods to choose from.
- **PUNGENT** cares for the Lung and Large Intestine—yellow onions (cooked), garlic, ginger (not always bladder-safe), radish, Chinese chives (cooked), black/white pepper, spicy peppers (may not be tolerated), cayenne (LaJiao), liquor, etc.
- **BITTER** cares for the Heart and Small Intestine—kale (GanLanCai), lettuce, dandelion (PuGongYing), broccoli, arugula (ZhiMaCai), endive (JuJuCai), collard greens (LvganLan), kernel (Ku Xing Ren), ginkgo biloba (Bai Guo), leaf of lycium fruit (Gou Qi Ye), biota leaf (Ce Bai Ye), peach kernel (Tao Ren), prepared soybean (Dan Dou Chi), lotus leaves (Lian Ye), mugwort leaf (Ai Ye), liquor, pig liver, etc. Many of these foods have not been tested by IC/BPS patients, so sticking with the foods you are familiar with is wise.

- **SALTY** nourishes the Kidney and Bladder—kelp or seaweed (HaiDai), laver (ZiCai, which is a sea plant), cuttlefish bone (Hai Piao Xiao), oyster, sea blubber (Hai Zhe), octopus, pig kidney, pig foot, salt, etc.

Many other foods are typically listed under the different properties, but some of the previous list has been modified to meet the IC/BPS diet guidelines.

The color of a food plays a role in food energies, as does the doctrine of signatures (the other properties). Green foods cherish the liver. Red food adores the heart. Yellow food esteems the spleen. White food loves the lung and black food adores the kidney.

A bitter green like kale will nourish the heart because of its bitter property and will cherish the liver because of its green color. It will also nourish the kidney, and especially the bones, because of its rich minerals. (Kale should be included in the diet to help prevent osteoporosis.)

Red foods, such as red peppers, usually nourish the heart and small intestine. The apple nourishes the spleen and the kidney because of its sweet property when it is baked and lightly salted. Of course, many IC/BPS patients cannot tolerate apples.

White foods like white onions and tofu (which usually must be avoided to prevent IC/BPS symptoms) nourish the lung and large intestine, while the radish (which may also need to be avoided) assists the liver because its pungent property helps to move stagnant Qi (energy) out of the liver. Some detoxifying drinks contain radish.

This information on Chinese Medicine was written with the assistance of Dr. Wen Xuan (wenxuan@hotmail.com). Chinese medical treatments may take a few weeks to take effect. A combination of acupuncture and herbal medicine usually works the fastest, and acupuncture is probably the most bladder-friendly of the three Chinese treatments.

Mind/Body and Pain Management Programs

Most urologists and urogynecologists who treat IC/BPS know all too well how challenging it can be for patients to get to their appointments, not to mention commit to classes or programs. But when patients see specialists for their overlapping conditions, such as FMS, migraine headaches, or temporomandibular disorder (TMJD), these specialists may refer them to pain management or wellness programs. However, what they may not realize is that IC/BPS patients might be hesitant about attending classes with others who do not have a bladder disease. This is not to say that these programs aren't helpful to chronic pain patients, because they are. Mind/body, wellness, and pain management programs are designed to help chronic pain patients with coping strategies such as relaxation and guided imagery, cognitive restructuring (modifying one's response to her/his painful and troublesome symptoms), behavior therapy, practical lifestyle modifications, group therapy, exercise, and sometimes nutrition management. These programs are designed to empower individuals and provide them with a feeling of control and success.

Although most patients are encouraged to participate at their own pace, IC/BPS patients might need to make even more modifications for their specific needs. The following suggestions may be helpful and some can be used in place of the instructed methods:

- MODIFICATIONS FOR COMFORT—When you begin a program, let your facilitator know if you have frequency and need to sit near a door to leave without interruption. Bring a cushion for sitting or back support. You will usually be given the option to bend your knees when lying down.
- MODIFICATIONS FOR EXERCISE—Use your own judgment when asked to take certain positions or perform certain exercises. Some of the positions and slow motions of movement rituals such as yoga or Tai Chi may be too demanding; however, a facilitator will usually offer alternative options for individual needs. If you need to skip an

exercise, try to do so without interrupting, and then talk to your facilitator after class about your future needs.

- NUTRITION MANAGEMENT—Eating is thought to release endorphins, which make us feel better. Learning good nutrition and how foods can help to fight pain is very important; however, some foods such as those that elevate serotonin levels may help FMS patients but cause bladder pressure, pain, and frequency in IC/BPS patients. *Refer to Chapter Two for nutritional information.*

- BREATHING MODIFICATIONS—Techniques such as mindful breathing use diaphragmatic breathing, which focuses on movement in the belly. Diaphragmatic breathing is very important to IC/BPS and FMS patients, because it helps to slow the sympathetic nervous system and stretch tight muscles. It also helps patients who do not breathe fully due to pain. However, not all IC/BPS patients can comfortably focus on and breathe into their bellies without stirring bladder pressure, pain, or frequency. Instead, IC/BPS patients can produce the same helpful results by focusing their breath and movement into their ribs: front, sides, and back. (Three dimensional breathing is another Aston-Patterning concept.)

Relaxation and Visualization Exercises

Although this may come as no surprise to IC/BPS patients, unlike other muscles of the body, the pelvic floor muscles never rest. This makes perfect sense to patients who have difficulty getting these muscles to relax after a flare-up caused by stress. These patients know that managing stress is essential to keep symptoms at bay. However, relaxation or guided imagery exercises that require patients to focus on their sites of pain in order to relax, or imagine the healing process taking place, are not usually as successful for IC/BPS patients as distraction exercises are. So, instead of focusing on the bladder, patients can try focusing on the sacral area (the flat triangular bone at the bottom of the spine), the tail bone, and the perineal area (between the anus and vagina or testes) to achieve relaxation. Reintroducing movement and feeling to other areas of the body that are tense and painful due to the referred pain of IC/BPS, is often helpful.

> *According to Jerome Weiss, M.D., stress can pull the coccyx (tail bone) forward, compressing the organs that run through the pelvic floor muscles and pulling them up against the pubic bone. This physical reaction to stress, plus the release of histamine and other inflammatory agents, trigger IC/BPS symptoms in patients.*

When techniques and relaxation exercises are used to decrease the stress and fears that accompany IC/BPS, they can help calm and control the illness. Practicing relaxation daily encourages the healing process in both the body and mind. One wonderful stress management technique is called **Focusing**, which was created by Gene Gendlin in the 1960s. Focusing is especially helpful to deal with worries or problems that don't seem manageable. With regular practice, relief is experienced in the body. It is best to begin with the instruction of someone else's voice.

Focusing

- Start by closing your eyes. Take a few cleansing breaths and imagine that you are stepping back from your problems for a while.
- Picture a place like a beach or park, a beautiful and comfortable place in nature, a place that feels safe. Wherever it is, it is a place where you will be able to empty your bladder comfortably if needed. You are in total control. Find a comfortable place to sit and take in the beauty of this place.
- Sense the temperature, the smells, the sounds of the birds, the wind in the trees or the surf. You feel very peaceful in this special place. Allow yourself to take it all in with no pressures to do anything or go anywhere.
- After you feel the comfort and serenity of this place, see if there is an issue or problem that has been in your way. If there is more than one problem, pick the biggest. Don't let yourself think about it, just pick it out.

- Now take this problem or a few problems if you cannot choose one, and place them away from you on a far rock, hill, or tree top.
- After you place your problem or line up your problems on a distant site, notice what comes into your feelings. Notice if there is anything else, maybe something that you did not consider as a problem right away, or something that you didn't consider so important. If there is something else, line it up on the distant site. Take a breath and make a choice, pick one issue, one that feels right or stands out for now.
- For a few moments feel what part of your body the problem affects—your gut, your shoulders? Once you feel the affected area imagine what your problem looks like. Does it have a color or colors? Do the colors (or color) fit the intensity or darkness of the problem? After you've given your problem colors, pick a shape for your problem. Is it round or long? Does this shape move? Notice how it feels in your body.
- Once you've visualized and experienced the problem in your body, place it back on that far site away from you. Take a few cleansing breaths and notice how you feel with your problem so far away.
- Picture yourself standing up, turning, and walking away, leaving the rock, hill, or tree top behind you. As you turn and walk away, take in the beauty of this very special place.
- When you are ready, slowly open your eyes and take a little time to stretch and focus your eyes. Notice how you feel. Perhaps you feel lighter, more relaxed, and have a different perspective than before this wonderful exercise.

Different variations of Focusing have been used over the years.

Post-Traumatic Stress Syndrome

Although it is beneficial to learn how to cognitively deal with a flare-up (modifying the response to pain to better cope with the situation), the pain of IC/BPS automatically induces an emotional response. Many theorists, both traditional and alternative, believe that chronic pain patients often can't cope well with their pain because it brings up old traumas and unsafe feelings. In some instances this is true. For many IC/BPS patients the trauma of past negative, painful, and unproductive doctor visits and procedures have resulted in some post-traumatic stress. Nevertheless, the unique pain of IC/BPS causes behavior that is often misunderstood and mislabeled even by pain-management facilitators who claim they are experienced and familiar with the disease.

The pain of IC/BPS is carried to the center of the brain that carries emotion, and because IC/BPS affects an internal organ (the bladder), it is considered visceral pain. Visceral pain sends messages to the part of the brain called the limbic system, which regulates arousal and emotion. The messages from the bladder pain can make a patient feel upset, emotional, and depressed as a result. Patients may be seen as emotionally laden victims of a traumatic experience, demonstrating hyper-vigiliant behavior (the need to be on guard against harm), instead of a person in need of medication to treat the unsettling symptoms of IC/BPS. Because many IC/BPS patients are unable to sit still, relax, or focus on their bladder pain (in a wellness program), they may be misjudged. It is important for patients to discuss this issue with a pain-management program facilitator to avoid being misunderstood.

Compulsions, quirks, or eccentric behaviors that exist before IC/BPS will stand a chance of being magnified during flare-ups. And, it is not unusual for IC/BPS patients to experience their first symptoms of IC/BPS after a stressful event. Stress can trigger the symptoms of IC/BPS, but cannot in itself cause IC/BPS. Unfortunately, the type of behavior that IC/BPS pain sets off is similar to the type of behavior seen in patients with post-traumatic stress syndrome.

Many practitioners in both the alternative and traditional field continue to be guilty of misdiagnosing chronic pain patients as victims of stress. And when these patients do not get proper medical treatment, they can suffer and display enormous stress from being placed in this unfortunate situation. An unproductive, vicious cycle often results because these patients have been diagnosed and judged incorrectly.

After reading an article which lumped IC/BPS with other conditions defined as "somatic symptom syndrome" (unexplained by identifiable disease even after extensive medical assessment), IC/BPS patient Rachel Fazio, M.S., P.L.P.C., decided to do a small study on 48 IC/BPS patients. Rachel used the Minnesota Multiple Personality Inventory to demonstrate that IC/BPS patients are just like other legitimate chronic pain patients.

The result of her study turned out exactly as she had thought: The majority of patients in her study showed the kind of profile that correlates with people who have high-intensity and chronicity (long-lasting) pain, functional limitations (not being able to do everyday things), and poor response to medical treatment. "In other words," Rachel laments, "our psychological functioning is just like that of someone with a legitimate, conspicuous cause of chronic pain." Although a few patients' scores indicated that they were malingering (exaggerating their symptoms to get some kind of gain), Rachel states that "maybe these patients are having problems getting their doctors to listen to them and therefore have to complain more about their symptoms in order to get the treatment they need … who's not listening? So, to sum it up, the vast majority of us are not crazy. Either our psychological functioning is almost entirely normal, or just like that of a person with legitimate chronic pain. Maybe the problem lies in that the doctors that we deal with are not trained in chronic pain. In fact, based on these results, I would like to see IC/BPS patients get more involved with chronic pain doctors and comprehensive chronic pain clinics since the psychological profiles are so similar (to patients with high-intensity and chronicity pain) and that sort of treatment helps so many people with chronic pain."

In a *Time* magazine article written in 2005, called "Why Don't More Docs Get It Right," Dr. Scott Fishman of U.C. Davis complained, "If comprehensive pain-management centers are so good at providing relief, why aren't more doctors following their lead?" Fishman clearly recognized that most doctors don't understand chronic pain: "We don't teach medical students enough about pain, even though it's the most common reason people go to doctors."

Perhaps, if more doctors were trained in chronic pain management, they would understand their patients' behavior and the trickle-down effect of this understanding would eventually enable more nurses, therapists, technicians, and other health-care practitioners, both traditional and alternative, to understand too. In the meantime, IC/BPS patients, along with the IC/BPS associations, networks and institutions, must continue to educate health-care providers.

Pain specialist, who believe IC/BPS is a psychological disorder still exist!

Resources

Aston-Patterning Training Center
P.O. Box 3568 • Incline Village, NV 89450
www.astonkinetics.com • (775) 831-8228

Upledger Institute International (Craniosacral treatment)
11211 Prosperity Farms Rd., Suite D-325
Palm Beach Gardens, FL 33410
www.upledger.com • (800) 233-5880

American Academy of Medical Acupuncture (Patient referral line)
www.medicalacupuncture.org • (310) 364-0193

Books

The Better Bladder Book, Wendy Cohan, R.N.

IC Naturally, Diana Brady, M.A., C.N.C.

Chapter Five

COPING WITH NEW PRESCRIPTIONS, DOCTORS, AND SENSITIVITIES TO MEDICATIONS

As with different foods, certain medications can trigger interstitial cystitis/bladder pain syndrome and other painful bladder syndromes. The idea that so many drugs can have such an effect on the bladder is hard for many doctors to accept.

Although individual patients have different susceptibilities to drugs, most IC/BPS patients have experienced a bladder flare-up after taking a particular medication. According to IC/BPS surveys, a large percentage of IC/BPS patients suffer with sensitivities or severe allergic reactions to medications. Even so, there is little documentation and not much known about the side effects medications and their fillers, coatings, and capsules can produce in IC/BPS patients. It still rests with the individual to determine which medications trigger bladder symptoms and/or allergic reactions.

The following is not intended to augment the information given to patients by their own doctors; however, most doctors do not understand IC/BPS and find chronic pain patients, in general, difficult to treat. It's not unusual for IC/BPS patients to have to search out the right doctors in order to receive appropriate medications and treatments without side effects. This especially applies to patients living in small towns and rural areas where there are no large medical communities.

Trial by Error

Dealing with New Doctors

When seeing a new doctor or specialist for a problem other than IC/BPS, patients don't know if the physician will be receptive to their IC/BPS needs. Specialists, after all, are interested in treating the condition that they are being consulted for. Bladder disease is not their main concern and a patient's knowledge about her or his body may be dismissed. Even when seeking treatment for an overlapping condition, such as fibromyalgia (FMS), a sympathetic specialist familiar with chronic pain patients may not understand or agree with IC/BPS pain management. As a matter of fact, doctors who specialize in newly researched diseases often have opinions as to the cause and treatment for conditions that support their theories and specialties. One extreme example is the number of psychiatrists who believe that IC/BPS is the result of sexual abuse and/or a psychiatric disorder.

Feeling challenged in the doctor's office is still a common experience for most women. Sadly, this circumstance disempowers patients, causes emotional pain, and sometimes results in physical pain. IC/BPS patients may become so discouraged by such negative experiences that they give up on treatments and medications that may help them. Some patients just settle for pain or other conditions that might be treatable, or relieved by the right doctor who will work with their needs.

Fortunately, there are doctors who evaluate the success of treatments for chronic pain patients differently than for the average population. This is so important to the many IC/BPS patients who are sensitive, do not respond quickly to treatments, cannot fit into standard treatment agendas, and/or have mutifactorial pain (different sources of pain). However, on occasion doctors may choose not to treat sensitive patients in order to avoid hurting them. Or, patients may not get treatment when doctors who do not know how to treat them speak in a clinical manner to hide their ignorance. And also there are doctors who are afraid of being sued by patients who list many allergies and drug sensitivities. It is necessary to understand these dynamics to avoid useless, repeated visits to doctors who cannot help.

Qualities that Make a Good Doctor
- A doctor who listens
- A doctor who accepts the fact that any medication may cause an adverse reaction in your body, although there is little documentation and not much known about the side effects medications and their fillers can produce in IC/BPS patients
- A doctor you feel comfortable calling when a drug has an adverse reaction in your bladder or elsewhere. Not letting a doctor know gives him or her the impression that the drug worked. This won't help you or other IC/BPS patients.
- A doctor who understands that you must be cautious when trying a new medication
- A doctor who will not challenge you or try to fit you into the profile of standard medical care
- A doctor who will never compare you to another IC/BPS patient
- A doctor who is not threatened by your knowledge of IC/BPS and related conditions
- A doctor who doesn't label you or make you feel neurotic when you explain your physical problems
- A doctor (urologist or urogynecologist) who will give you a "rescue instillation" when you need one

When seeing a doctor who usually has you sitting in the waiting room for over half an hour, call the office ahead of your appointment to see if he/she is running late. If the doctor is behind, ask when you should arrive for your appointment.

Bring an Advocate to Your Doctor Visit

New doctors usually respond well to patients who bring along an advocate. An advocate is someone who can back you up, someone who has experience with your condition and can remember important things that you may forget. Any grown person can be your advocate—a partner, a parent, an aunt or uncle, cousin or friend. Older children can also act as advocates for their parents. All said, Daniel Brookoff, M.D., honestly suggested that patients who bring along an adult white male will usually be more validated by a doctor. This is sad, but often true.

When new patients are afraid to ask for support from others, they most likely haven't learned how to self-advocate. Depending on personality and past medical experiences, learning to be your own advocate is usually a process. Recognizing the importance of self-advocacy, Molly Hanna Glidden, former support group leader of the Boston MetroWest IC Support Group, created five proactive steps for patients:

1. Always trust your instincts and good judgment. Tap your inner wisdom when dealing with others, especially doctors.
2. Research everything! Learning about IC/BPS and the available treatment options will help you to discuss your health issues with a doctor. Keep in mind that a doctor is working for you.
3. Join a support group to find valuable guidance and friendly support. Sharing with other patients is an important step toward self-advocacy, because it can help you to feel less isolated and more empowered. Networking with other patients to find doctors is another bonus.
4. Speak up and get your needs met. Sometimes family and friends cannot relate to IC/BPS; perhaps because it is an invisible disease. Don't let this stop you from letting others know your limitations. If you cannot educate them with conversation, leave IC/BPS articles and pamphlets around your home or workplace where people can see them and read them. Printed information legitimizes your condition.
5. Take positive action on your "good days." Do things that make you happy. Visit a favorite spot or buy something special, just for yourself. Actions like these will keep your mind and body moving in a positive direction.

Learning to self-advocate usually doesn't take long because the symptoms of IC/BPS demand lifestyle changes. Contrary to what some may believe, other people admire patients who stand up for themselves to get their needs met. Still, bringing an advo-cate to a new doctor visit adds validation.

Communicating with New Doctors

Doctors sometimes have difficulty with anxious patients, but the very nature of IC/BPS naturally makes patients anxious. Bad experiences with doctors and medications also lead to anxiety. Therefore practicing a sense of control, by staying as calm as possible and giving a doctor a chance to understand you, can help you get what you need. Feeling a sense of control in the of-fice may also mean taking a practice drive or train ride to a new doctor's office in order to know what you can expect logistically. Some patients find afternoon appointments less stressful since the bladder is more active in the morning and a decent night's sleep, which may include sleeping into the later morning hours, can make all the difference.

Trying a New Prescription

Prescription drugs and their fillers, the inert ingredients in medications, go through the body in different ways. Both syn-thetic and natural medications can affect different parts of the central nervous system and cause allergic reactions. This is no surprise to the many IC/BPS patients who experience drug reac-tions and sensitivities in their bladders as well as in other areas of their bodies. The side effects to the central nervous system and the atypical reactions of many IC/BPS patients make trying a new drug difficult and often frightening.

Consulting a *Physicians Desk Reference*, or the *Pharmacist's Guide to Over-the-Counter and Natural Remedies* on-line, and/or becoming friendly with a pharmacist can be helpful and some-times necessary in order to find information about drug fillers, coatings, and capsules used in medications, documented drug interactions, and side effects. A knowledgeable pharmacist can also direct a patient to a formulating or compounding pharmacy, which may be able to tailor a prescription to the individual's needs or offer natural sources, which may be better tolerated than synthetic ones. A pharmacist can offer information on alternative options to oral medications, such as topical creams, ointments, skin patches, and liquid medications (that often contain less additives). The most valuable information, however, may come from another IC/BPS patient with similar symptoms. After all, it was an IC/BPS patient who first alerted a doctor about what hurt her or his bladder. It was a good doctor who researched the reason and informed other patients and doctors.

When you are unsure of a newly prescribed medication, ask the pharmacist for only three pills to begin with (you may want to pay in cash instead of using your insurance). Explain to your doctor and your pharmacist that you will fill the whole prescription if the medication doesn't trigger your IC/BPS symptoms or other reactions. If you are very sensitive to medications, you can ask your doctor or pharmacist if it's possible to begin with a quarter or half dose and gradually increase to full dosage. But, always check if a tablet can be cut or a capsule can be emptied into water before ingesting. Some medications have enteric coating (such as time-released medicines) or are put into capsules to avoid direct contact with the stomach. (Patients should not take antacids or drink milk with pills with enteric coating. Capsules can be taken with a hot drink to make them dissolve and go to work faster.) Let your doctor know that you understand the small amount is not therapeutic, not enough to treat the condition, but that this is a necessary experiment for your bladder and other sensitivities. If you usually experience a cumulative effect, and don't experience IC/BPS symptoms until a few days or weeks after taking a new medication, inform your doctor that you may not know if you can tolerate the medication right away.

Contents from capsules must be stirred well if the medication is time released. One or two sips should be enough to detect a problem. Teaching hospitals may have formulating pharmacies for patients.

If You Have a Bad Reaction

Always let a doctor know if a drug has an adverse effect on your bladder or elsewhere. Although you may not want to deal with a doctor after a problem, you give your doctor the false impression that you improved with the prescribed treatment if you do not let him or her know otherwise. The doctor may also possibly make the same mistake with another IC/BPS patient.

It is also very important to report adverse drug reactions to the drug companies because they record adverse reactions. Medications that list urinary retention, urinary frequency and/ or bladder pain, bladder infections, difficulty with urination, leg pain, and other similar side effects in their inserts send out a red flag to IC/BPS patients. Drugs with these listed side effects may easily trigger IC/BPS symptoms. Even so, some specialists will tell you that almost all medications list urinary side effects, so it doesn't really mean anything significant. But, these side effects are significant and real. They have been reported and should be considered before taking a new medication.

Because new medications can present challenges, the IC/BPS patient isn't always considered a so called "good patient," and some doctors can make the IC/BPS patient feel indulgent and neurotic. When this occurs, it's best to try to find another doctor. Although it takes time, energy, and often courage to regroup before a new doctor search, the IC/BPS patient need not continue to be victimized by the disease *and* the wrong doctor.

Joy Selak, Ph.D., IC/BPS patient, and co-author with Steven S. Overman, M.D., of *You Don't Look Sick,* adheres to a "three strikes and you're out" rule with doctors. Joy came up with this sensible rule when she was seeking a good health-care partner. She also notes the traits necessary for a mutual patient/physician relationship:

- We must treat each other with courtesy.
- We must see each other as unique.
- We must make our responses to each other as honest and informed and respectful as we possibly can.
- We must be willing to work together to build trust.

Surgeries and Hospital Stays

Dealing with surgeries and hospital stays can be very difficult for IC/BPS patients. Although it may not always be possible, it's helpful to be fully prepared before going into the hospital for surgery or certain treatments. Preparation is especially important for those who have experienced bad reactions to drugs or those with multiple chemical sensitivity (MCS).

Patients who are undergoing surgery (not emergency) have the opportunity to talk to the anesthesiologist in advance about existing drug sensitivities. The doctor may take an interest and work with them individually. Patients who are particularly sensitive to drugs may want to also contact Dr. Ann McCampbell of the Multiple Chemical Sensitivities Task Force of New Mexico. Dr. McCampbell can provide information for sources of preservative-free medications and other products for sensitive patients. *See Resources.*

Although it is helpful to avoid certain medications, it may still be impossible to avoid bladder irritation. Many IC/BPS patients have overlapping conditions and require pre-operative medications and medications during surgery that can irritate the bladder. Therefore, it is important to plan and consider what pain management can be used after surgery to reduce pain from a procedure, as well as pain caused by the adverse effects of medications.

Another consideration can occur when an IV saline drip is used. Potassium is sometimes added to the saline solution and should be avoided. Patients need to notify the doctor of this problem, because potassium is a known bladder irritant for IC/ BPS patients.

After surgery some IC/BPS patients find hydrocodone or a shot of morphine (a morphine drip doesn't always address bladder pain) effective for pain, including bladder pain. Another pain medication option is tramadol (Ultram), but not all IC/BPS patients can tolerate tramadol. Patients who use heat or ice for pain may need to order hot or cold packs before surgery.

Since IC/BPS patients often experience urinary frequency after surgery, it is important to plan ahead. Depending on a nurse to come in frequently with a bedpan is unrealistic. Plus, bedpans aren't very sturdy and are not meant for constant use. The best solution may be a potty chair placed beside the bed, or patients who do not have adverse reactions to catheters might ask to be catheterized for surgery and hospital recovery. This procedure can help rid irritating urine. However, most doctors don't like to use catheters on short surgeries and usually use adult catheters on adults. When doctors would prefer not to use a pediatric catheter, which is smaller and more comfortable, patients can ask for adult-size catheters, "12" or "14." These are small adult sizes. It's necessary that the nurse knows to check the urine bag often after surgery. It will probably fill up more quickly than the average patient's. When it gets too full, urine can back up, creating unnecessary discomfort and pain for even the average patient.

Even with a catheter, some patients feel the need to void naturally after surgery. With the doctor's consent, the nurse can remove the catheter and help the patient to a potty chair. Bedpans are very awkward for female IC/BPS patients. Nurses expect patients to sit in the middle of the bed but IC/BPS patients do best when they sit on the side of the bed with their feet on the floor. However, it usually takes two people to maneuver this position.

Avoiding air pollution in the hospital room can be another challenge to IC/BPS patients in an emergency hospitalization. Those who are sensitive to odors and fumes can ask in advance, if possible, for a hospital room that has not been newly disinfected, painted or carpeted, or sprayed with pesticides. While in the hospital, housekeeping can be informed not to use strong disinfectants or cleaning products. If the hospital stay is short, it may be best not to have the room cleaned. Although nurses and assistants are usually taught in their training to avoid wearing perfume while on duty, many do not comply with this suggestion. Perfume and scented laundry detergent worn by caretakers are a problem for sensitive patients, and it is not always easy to get hospital staff to listen. Most hand sanitizers can also irritate sensitive patients and the majority of staff who walk into the hospital room will immediately pump the dispenser on the wall. Wearing a mask when needed may be necessary. Being able to open a window is not always an option.

Another very important consideration for patients is dietary management. Patients who must follow a diet for IC/BPS can talk to the hospital dietitian and plan meals before the hospital stay. But, it can be difficult or sometimes impossible to get plain foods, such as a soft boiled egg or a baked potato, because many hospitals contract with outside vendors and have limited internal resources. A liquid diet can also bring a challenge because most of the liquids will be citrus and so will the sherbet and popsicles. Arranging to have meals brought in may be necessary. Although a microwave and refrigerator are typically available for patient use, it is unrealistic to expect hospital staff to warm meals or bring snacks. A partner, friend, private sitter, or certified nursing assistant may be needed the first day or so.

> *Most hospitals provide meals that are processed and unhealthy, but the Cleveland Clinic in Ohio has tried to change this trend. The Clinic and the Clinic's sister hospitals are promoting healthy practices and prevention for employees, patients, and their families, which includes serving healthy foods. Even though healthy food doesn't always equal bladder-friendly food, it's good to know that hospitals are starting to pay attention to the foods they serve.*

Coping with General Conditions, Routine Exams, and Procedures Without the Drugs and Fillers That Might Trigger IC/BPS Pain

Commonly used medications, as well as certain medical diagnostic exams and routine procedures, can present a challenge to IC/BPS patients. Medications that are used for general conditions may trigger bladder pain. These include acid-blocking and antiulcer medications, antibiotics, some anti-inflammatory medications, anti-nausea medications, cough medicines, epinephrine and other decongestants and stimulants, laxatives, muscle relaxants, and stool softeners. Many inactive ingredients in medications can also trigger bladder pain and other sensitivities. Magnesium is one additive that may adversely affect IC/BPS patients.

Magnesium is used in a number of medications and is known to be a bladder irritant. Another inactive ingredient, propylene glycol (found in certain medicines such as some medications to treat yeast infections), may also trigger bladder symptoms.

IC/BPS patients who experience skin rashes and digestive problems with oral antidepressants and pain medications may be helped by using a formulating pharmacy. Antidepressants and pain gels can be formulated for topical use. But there's a draw-back; they often are not as effective as oral medication, and usually must be applied a few times a day.

Information and options in this chapter are intended only as suggestions and should be discussed with your doctor.

Dental Visits

An array of different chemicals and materials (including latex or vinyl gloves) are used in the dentist office. One of the biggest culprits for the IC/BPS patient is epinephrine. Epinephrine is used in injections, inhalers, eye drops, and nose drops (and also during surgeries). Epinephrine is added to the numbing agent in the injection given before an invasive dental procedure. Epinephrine will affect the tone of the bladder and may cause IC/BPS symptoms. Patients can ask the dentist to skip the epinephrine. The numbing agent may be short lived without epinephrine and an additional injection may be required, but this is usually more tolerable than experiencing IC/BPS pain during or after a dental procedure. Some IC/BPS patients, however, are also sensitive to certain numbing agents. Patients with multiple chemical sensitivity (MCS) may experience sensitivity to numbing agents too. Trying alternative agents may be necessary.

Other substances used during crown work can trigger bladder pain and chemical sensitivity. If you have experienced problems after crown work, ask your dentist or surgeon for an ion temporary crown instead of an acrylic one, and for non-eugenol cement (made by Proviscell). Let your dentist or surgeon know if glues, astringents, or bleaches are irritating so he or she will work closely with you to find alternatives, such as using saline solution instead of bleach when possible. Also ask your dentist or surgeon if you can avoid a medicated pack with your temporary crown. Although an antibacterial agent may be necessary, if it can safely be avoided, you may avoid bladder pain.

Odors from glues and cements used during crown work can be overwhelming. A hand-held fan can help to minimize the noxious fumes.

IC/BPS patients with mitral valve prolapse (MVP) often have another problem when they are advised to take an antibiotic before invasive dental work. (Those with joint replacements also are advised to take an antibiotic before dental work.) Patients who cannot tolerate oral antibiotics without bladder pain may instead try an antibiotic drip before dental work. This may require the help of your primary care doctor. (Of course, even some antibiotic drips can affect the bladder.) It is very important that IC/BPS patients with MVP work closely with primary care doctors. Some patients with very mild MVP are told by doctors that an antibiotic is not necessary; however, patients having major dental work may want to consult their doctors first.

Dental work can often irritate the bladder no matter how well pain prevention has been practiced. It's also not unusual for some IC/BPS patients to experience prolonged pain and inflammation in their teeth after a procedure. This condition, however, does not mean that IC/BPS patients should not have the dentist or oral surgeon double-check their dental work.

Patients who would like to know their sensitivities to agents and materials used in dental work may contact Clifford Consulting and Research. These consultants provide Materials Reactivity Testing. Refer to Resources.

Eye Exams, Solutions, and Drops

Not many patients are aware that what goes into their tear ducts goes into their system. Patients who are sensitive to epinephrine might avoid bladder pain and other reactions by asking their doctors to leave the epinephrine out of the dilating drops used during a routine eye exam. Although the epinephrine enables the drops to last longer, a routine eye exam will usually work fine without the use of epinephrine.

Eye drops in general contain medicines, preservatives, and stabilizers that may irritate the IC/BPS bladder. Eye medications are often available in both drops and ointments, and ointments seem to be less irritating. However, if drops are necessary a patient can lie down, place her/his thumb and middle finger on the inside corner of her/his eye, and apply gentle pressure for five minutes after applying each drop. Following these instructions can help to block medications from draining through the duct and causing side effects. Of course, with any new eye medication it's important to begin with the lowest dose.

Sensitive IC/BPS patients who wear contact lens may not realize that contact cleaning solutions can contain bladder irritants. For instance, some patients can't tolerate boric acid. Experimenting by wearing glasses instead of contacts for a few days may indicate if a solution is triggering IC/BPS symptoms. Patients who suffer with dry eyes may find they have a reaction to commercial brands of saline solution. Some patients may, however, tolerate Refresh Tears which is found in drug stores. Alternative brands of eye drops are available at health food stores or shops that sell natural remedies. Some of these brands are homeopathic and a small amount can be very strong and sometimes irritating. To identify which drops are irritating, try brands with the fewest ingredients and use only a small drop in one eye to begin with.

Bronchodilator Inhaler

Inhalers used to treat asthma often contain epinephrine and other stimulating chemicals that can affect bladder function in IC/BPS patients, as well as cause other unpleasant reactions in those with chemical sensitivity. IC/BPS patients with respiratory problems may have to use a steroid inhaler to avoid bladder spasms. (There may be some patients who are sensitive to steroid inhalers.) Although inhaled steroids work preventively with long-term use and are not intended for the short-term treatment of an asthma attack, they can work quickly to reduce histamines in a respiratory response to chemicals and irritants. However, patients with MCS often report difficulty with inhalers. Patients may do better with cromolyn inhalers. Treatments must be discussed with a doctor, preferably one who understands and believes that sensitivities are real and *organic* (caused by a physiological malfunction).

Antibiotics

Probably the most difficult drugs for IC/BPS patients are antibiotics. Antibiotic use was once suspected as being a cause of IC/BPS. Although this theory is usually no longer considered valid, many patients have taken a lot of antibiotics, and antibiotics often trigger IC/BPS flare-ups. Unfortunately, there's not much information available on this problem, and there are still doctors who have difficulty understanding or even treating patients who are sensitive to antibiotics.

The antibiotic Ciprofloxacin is sometimes prescribed for patients who are allergic to other antibiotics. This strong antibiotic may or may not be bladder-safe for all IC/BPS patients, although there has been speculation that Cipro (ciprofloxacin) and other fluoroquinolones might contain pain relieving properties. Leviquin (levofloxacin) is another antibiotic in this class that patients may tolerate, but patients should be aware that there are possible side effects of both antibiotics. Ciprofloxin and Leviquin can cause tendons to rupture; therefore, patients are advised to monitor exercise during treatment and for a period of time after treatment.

If a patient doubts the need for a prescribed antibiotic, a doctor can be asked to check, if possible, to see if there's a bacterial infection. When antibiotics are necessary, the doctor should be able to work with a patient to prescribe one that is fairly bladder-safe. However, depending on the infection, at some point an IC/BPS patient may require an antibiotic that is irritating. Some patients find that they have less reaction in their bladders when antibiotics are given intravenously (this procedure may not be covered by insurance) or taken in one mega-dose if possible, but this is not always the case.

Pain medications may be necessary when taking irritating antibiotics. Patients who use antidepressants to treat their IC/BPS may find it helpful to take a very small amount of an antidepressant when pain occurs. (Of course, it's necessary to be cautious when taking a drug during the day which is usually intended for use at night.) Another way to fight breakthrough bladder pain is with a bladder instillation containing a numbing agent or a prescribed topical pain gel. Although combination pain gels containing more than one medicine are often helpful, IC/BPS patients should try one ingredient at a time.

Antibiotics can set off more than bladder symptoms. They can cause vaginal yeast infections, especially in women with IC/BPS, and women with other chronic conditions and autoimmune conditions. Antibiotics can also trigger stomach problems and an array of reactions in sensitive patients. Therefore, it's necessary to take probiotics while on antibiotics and continue taking them up to a month after stopping antibiotics. Ideally, patients should take tolerated probiotics every day.

Preventing Yeast Infections

Women with compromised immune systems (which may or may not be the case in individual IC/BPS patients) are prone to yeast infections, but both the medication to treat yeast and the yeast infection itself can irritate the bladder. Therefore, it's always necessary to use prevention. Wear only 100 percent cotton panties (preferably organic cotton). Sprinkle a little corn starch, which is usually bladder-friendly, in your panties and change them if they become damp or moist. (Avoid corn starch that has been genetically modified—look for the GMO Free logo.) If tight panties irritate your bladder and vulva, try Long-Torso Comfort Briefs which can be ordered from the Vermont Country Store. Use only non-conventional, unscented brands of soaps and detergents (found at health food stores and some grocery stores). It's also important to avoid conventional and scented brands of fabric softeners. Cleanse the vaginal area both morning and night, and change towels daily. Avoid tampons, or use the smallest size, and ideally, change after each urination (which is usually impossible so instead, change often). Even though it's necessary to avoid scented protection, you may still be sensitive to the synthetic materials in conventional sanitary pads and tampons. Look for natural pads at the health food store or use washable GladRags, which are also found at most health food stores. When using an ice pack while traveling in a hot car, be sure to remove it as soon as it begins to melt. At home, wear dresses or skirts without underwear. Always avoid tight pants or synthetic leggings. Tight pants and leggings create a posterior pelvic position which pulls the pelvis back and under, increasing pressure on the sacrum (the triangular bone at the bottom of the spine where bladder nerves innervate).

Keep sugar and dairy intake moderate (except non-sugary yogurt if tolerated) and follow the IC/BPS diet. Patients find that eliminating yeast from their diets prevents both yeast infections and IC/BPS symptoms. The friendly bacteria found in probiotics can also prevent the constipation of irritable bowel syndrome (IBS). Because yeast flourishes in the large bowel during constipation, a bout of follow-up diarrhea can result in a yeast infection. Even when IBS symptoms aren't severe, yeast overgrowth may occur. But which probiotics are bladder-friendly? Again, tolerance is individual, but trying the lowest dose is almost always necessary. Klaire Labs Pro-Biotic Complex, mentioned in Chapter One under "Irritable Bowel Syndrome," is an excellent choice if tolerated. But, when patients have trouble with probiotics, they can try a mild, children's acidophilus. Of course, all IC/BPS patients should avoid acidophilus that contains aspartame, which is a bladder irritant.

Opinions differ as to when to take a probiotic. Patients can refer to the manufacturer's advice or their doctor's advice.

Although some experts advise patients to avoid yeast-fermented foods such as aged cheese, soy sauce, and pickles, there are a few probiotic foods that you may tolerate. If you can eat plain or vanilla yogurt, try Greek yogurt. The live active cultures L. Bulgaricus and S. Thermophilus in Greek yogurt help to prevent intestinal and vaginal imbalance. Choose Greek yogurt made from sheep's milk if you cannot tolerate cow's milk. (Yogurt contains bacteria that help to digest lactose.)

Vinegar-free pickles and sauerkraut provide a good source of lactobacillus. Bubbies make vinegar-free pickles and sauerkraut, but Bubbies pickles are a little spicy and have a kick. Bubbies vinegar-free sauerkraut is mild and has no heat. Ba-Tampte Half Sour Pickles contain no vinegar and aren't spicy except they do contain a lot of garlic. (Both Bubbies and Ba-Tampte pickles can be found at some Whole Foods Markets.) Cucumbers in brine also contain lactobacillus and are typically vinegar-free. Lowell Foods makes mild cucumbers in brine. *Refer to Resources.*

Long-torso cotton underwear can be ordered from The Vermont Country Store. See Resources. Some patients like panties made of bamboo and organic cotton (bluecanoe.com). (Patients should avoid underwear with antibacterial linings and anti-microbial finishes.)

Treating Yeast Infections

Vaginal creams used to treat yeast can create burning and spasms in patients with IC/BPS and vulvar vestibulitis. Vaginal creams may contain glycol propylene, alcohol, or sulfa which are often irritating to vaginal tissue. Some patients find they can tolerate a small amount at a time, about an inch of cream right before bed. Although this small amount may not work as quickly to cure a yeast infection, it's helpful to those who can tolerate it. Other patients may find it necessary to use medication only every other night. More than a few tubes of medication may be required to get rid of the infection. It's usually necessary for IC/BPS patients to keep the medication away from the urethra during insertion.

Another treatment option for yeast infections is Diflucan (fluconazole), an oral antifungal prescription drug. This medication is strong and needs to be prescribed and monitored by a doctor. Diflucan is not an optimal treatment for all IC/BPS patients, although it seems to be helpful to some patients with IC/BPS and vestibulitis who cannot use or get results with vaginal creams.

Mentioned before, probiotics, the live microorganisms similar to the good bacteria found in the gut, help digestion and elimination and prevent yeast from flourishing. Earth's Botanical Harvest makes Lactobacillus acidophilus Vaginal Suppositories that are usually bladder-safe and effective for many patients. (These suppositories must be inserted right before bed because they can melt quickly.) *See Resources.* Acidophilus capsules or powder (available at some health food stores) inserted with an applicator are also helpful to some patients.

Although soothing at first, yogurt inserted vaginally may cause bladder symptoms in some patients. Tough to treat yeast infections appear to respond to formulated boric acid, but sensitive IC/BPS patients may not tolerate boric acid very well and the use of boric acid is controversial.

The antifungal drug Nystatin is sometimes prescribed to treat stubborn yeast infections. This is a strong medication and has been reported to cause bladder symptoms in some IC/BPS patients.

Genital cultures may be needed to detect unusual species of yeast.

Treating Other Vaginal Infections

Bacterial vaginosis can require an antibacterial medicine such as the oral or vaginal cream Flagyl (metronidazole). Flagyl is a very strong drug and many IC/BPS patients have reactions in their bladders and elsewhere when they use it. Patients who find this drug intolerable should ask their doctor if they can be treated with the drug Cleocin (clindamycin) instead. Some IC/BPS patients seem to be able to tolerate Cleocin better than Flagyl. As always, treatment is very individual so it's best to be on the bladder-safe side and try vaginal creams a little at a time. Vaginal creams are usually better tolerated than vaginal gels which may have an alcohol base.

It's essential for IC/BPS patients to see a gynecologist when an infection is first suspected. Infections left untreated can become more difficult to treat and sometime require oral antibiotics. Always follow preventive measures.

Treating Stomach Problems

Certain medications and supplements, as well as medical conditions, can contribute to constipation. IC/BPS patients with irritable bowel syndrome (IBS), pelvic floor dysfunction (PFD), fibromyalgia (FMS), hypothyroidism, and other conditions often suffer with constipation. To compound this problem many medications to treat these conditions increase the likeliness of constipation. Pain medications, antidepressants, antacids, diuretics, and iron and calcium supplements all contribute to this problem.

Preventing constipation with diet is ideal, because taking fiber supplementation or drinks just adds more bulk to the existing bulk that occurs in patients with pelvic floor dysfunction and constipation IBS. Foods that are naturally high in fiber include cruciferous vegetables, such as broccoli, cauliflower, cabbage, and Brussels sprouts. These vegetables are also very good for people with allergies. According to nutrition expert Bonnie Minsky, "Some people with allergies have trouble removing toxins through the liver and kidneys." Minsky points out, "If the toxins back up into the body, it increases the chances of inflammation, which leaves an allergic person even more sensitive." Cruciferous vegetables also contain important antioxidants that counteract harmful free radicals that damage cells and DNA.

Constipation can also be somewhat relieved and prevented by using ground flaxseed or olive oil. (Flax seeds are very high in fiber and may not agree with some patients.) Olive oil is usually well tolerated by IC/BPS patients, is very healthy, and can be used generously on salads and vegetables. Eating brown rice or the seed quinoa for breakfast helps with motility of the digestive tract. Quinoa is a complete protein and is considered the least allergic seed. It is safe for patients with wheat, dairy, sugar, and gluten allergies or sensitivities, notes chef Lisa Williams (lisacookallergenfree.com). Sweet potatoes are also a good source of fiber and are high in vitamins C and B-6, as well as potassium. (Potassium in sweet potatoes does not seem to bother IC/BPS patients.) And a cup of lentils has six times more fiber than a daily serving of Metamucil. Figs are bladder-friendly for some patients and they too provide adequate fiber. Fig syrup, which is delicious, can be ordered from Barr.com.

According to the extended IC/BPS Food List, the fiber supplements that seem to be bladder-friendly are: acacia fiber, Benefiber, Metamucil (plain psyllium), and bulk psyllium (not sugar-free).

Relieving constipation can be very difficult for those with IBS, especially during perimenopause when estrogen wanes. Patients with constipation IBS should consider avoiding wheat and dairy products and follow a diet for IC/BPS as prevention. Since constipation can occur when B vitamin levels are low, patients must make an effort to eat foods that supply adequate amounts of these important vitamins. *See Chapter Two for more information on foods and the prevention and treatment of constipation and common diarrhea.*

Laxatives are often irritating to the IC/BPS bladder; however, over-the-counter MiraLax and Ducolax seem to be tolerated by some and can be used on occasion. Some IC/BPS who suffer with chronic constipation and/or IBS benefit from the prescription drug Amitiza (lubiprostone). According to the Fibromyalgia Network, fibromyalgia patients suffering with opiod-induced constipation have found relief with the drug Relistor, which is approved by the FDA for this problem with opioids. Relistor is an injectable medication and may not be appropriate for IC/BPS patients.

Some laxatives interfere with vitamin absorption. For instance, laxative mineral oil can dissolve the fat soluble vitamins A, D, and E. It's important that patients not become dependent on laxatives or stool softeners, especially those which irritate their bladders.

Cutting back on dairy products while taking laxatives may be necessary.

IC/BPS patients who suffer with constipation due to pelvic floor dysfunction should consider pelvic floor therapy to release the tight trigger points that prevent relaxation during elimination. Trigger points located in the abdominal muscles may also contribute to constipation. These too can be released for more comfort and easier elimination. Learning how to retrain muscles by engaging (contracting) the abdominal muscles while relaxing the sphincter (anus) muscle during elimination works well for many people. Though, at first it is a little like patting your head while rubbing your tummy.

Medications to stop diarrhea can trigger IC/BPS symptoms in some patients. Common diarrhea may be relieved with a few sips of slippery elm tea every half hour. Slippery elm soothes the membranes of the intestinal tract. Honey can be added to sweeten the tea. Although slippery elm is usually well tolerated by most IC/BPS patients, just two or three dunks of a tea bag or ball should be used. Eating a little barley, oat bran, or coconut macaroon cookies can also help control common diarrhea; however, barley green may irritate the bladder because of its high magnesium content. (Patients with celiac disease or gluten allergies must also avoid barley, macaroon cookies made with wheat flour, and oats that have been cross-pollenated with other grains.) American Saffron tea, made by Baar Products, can soothe the mucous membranes of the intestines after a bout of diarrhea and can be used daily to calm the colon. Another plus: some people have reported that the tea keeps their psoriasis at bay. The colon relates closely to the skin.

Replenish important minerals that are lost during diarrhea with a mineral rich broth. Combine:
3 quarts of spring water
2 zucchinis cut in big chunks
½ bunch celery
1 pack frozen green beans
Simmer for one hour (do not boil). Strain to remove the vegetables.

Suppositories, as well as other medications used to treat nausea, are not always bladder-safe. To relieve common nausea without drugs that might interfere with bladder function, try an old-fashioned remedy, Cola Syrup. A small amount mixed with non-carbonated water can help to relieve nausea. Cola Syrup (which does contain caffeine) can be ordered from The Vermont Country Store *(see Resources)* and appears to be bladder-safe for some patients.

Other alternative treatments for an unsettled stomach include a weak cup of chamomile, spearmint, peppermint, or ginger tea if tolerable. (Avoid herbal teas that contain caffeine.) Patients sensitive to herbs can try just one or two dunks of a tea bag or tea ball in hot water, and just a few sips of tea. Sometimes this is enough to help settle an upset stomach. IC/BPS patients who cannot tolerate peppermint tea may be able to drink spearmint tea. Plain mint teas are available through Celestial Seasonings found in health food stores and some conventional groceries. (Patients should avoid distilled water when they have diarrhea, flu, are vomiting, or when dehydrated.)

Acid reflux is a disorder that can accompany IBS. Reflux can also be caused by certain prescription drugs, but controlling reflux with acid-blocking medications (including Tagamet which is sometimes used to treat IC/BPS) has been known to irritate some patients' bladders. Over-the-counter acid-blocking products can also irritate the bladder because of the added preservatives used to further shelf life. Prevention, such as following a diet for IC/BPS, avoiding snacks before bedtime, and elevating the head of the bed four to six inches is usually the best approach to reduce common acid reflux.

Tums and Prelief can soothe the bladder and neutralize stomach acids that have an effect on esophageal reflux. IC/BPS patients, however, need to let doctors and pharmacists know if they are taking drugs or products that neutralize acidity, because the ingredients may interfere with the absorption of other drugs, including some of the drugs used to treat IC/BPS symptoms. Patients who take Tums are recommended to do so between meals.

Treating Allergies and Colds

Treating allergies with antihistamines can also relieve bladder symptoms in some patients. The drug hydroxyzine (Atarax and Vistaril) has been proven effective for the treatment of IC/BPS, allergies (not colds), migraines, and IBS thanks to the studies and interest of Dr. T. C. Theoharides and Dr. G. R. Sant. (Patients who are allergic to acacia should avoid Atarax which contains acacia.) But, it's very important for patients to understand that antihistamines containing decongestants can trigger IC/BPS symptoms. Patients who are sensitive to decongestants should avoid nose drops, sprays, and pills that contain decongestants. Although some IC/BPS patients find they are able to tolerate inhaled steroid sprays and some say they can actually tolerate small amounts of nasal sprays containing decongestants, others find they must treat nasal congestion with steam instead. Steam can actually be very effective when used two to three times a day. The easiest way to steam is to sit on a chair and lean over a sink of hot water (or over a pot of hot water) with a towel over your head. Drinking hot soups and weak teas (if possible) can also relax and open nasal passages.

> *Nasalcrom is another nasal spray option for sinus problems. It is also a treatment for IC/BPS.*

Other effective treatments for sinus relief, maintenance and prevention of allergies and colds include nasal rinsing, nasal ointment, and/or the Himalayan Salt Inhaler. Irrigating the nasal passages with baking soda and/or sea salt and water can be done with a syringe (ask your pharmacist) or with a Neti Pot. Those who do not like to pour water into their noses have the option of using the Himalayan Salt Inhaler, which also offers respiratory relief for asthma symptoms. (Asthma patients can experience flares when they have a bacterial imbalance in their intestines. Probiotics may be used as prevention.) A small amount of the nasal ointment Boroleum can as well be swabbed into the nostrils to relieve dry nasal tissue and prevent allergens and germs from entering the nasal passage. Boroleum is probably not safe for patients with multiple chemical sensitivity (MCS) because it contains camphor and menthol. It also may not be suitable for patients taking a homeopathic remedy. Boroleum and the Neti Pot can be ordered from The Vermont Country Store. The Neti Pot is also available at some Walgreen Drug Stores. The Himalayan Salt Inhaler can be ordered from Isabella. *See Resources.*

Although difficult to believe, some people claim that they avoid colds by wearing something called the Cold Coin. When worn on the body (preferably in the groin pocket) this coin, made of carbon steel, is meant to ionize the body with its vibrations to prevent and resist disturbances with the mucous membranes of the throat and nasal passages. Perhaps the power of positive thinking increases the benefits? The Cold Coin can be ordered from Baar. *See Resources.* Patients with mild IC/BPS symptoms may be able to maintain sinus health by rebounding on a mini trampoline. Of course, jumping up and down on a trampoline may be totally impossible for many patients, but some patients find they can do upper body exercises (without lifting their legs) successfully on a mini trampoline. The slight bounce created by the trampoline helps to tone the lower body.

It is best for patients to prevent sinus problems and allergies by modifying their environments, getting regular exercise and avoiding fermented foods, sugar, and dairy products that increase mucous. *Refer to Chapter Six to learn about environmental health.*

Certain healing properties in blueberries may actually help prevent allergies and most IC/BPS can eat these berries.

Sore throats and coughs that come with colds and flu can be soothed with warm saltwater gargles a few times a day. Antihistamines should be avoided. Popular cough drops may also have to be avoided, because they can set off bladder symptoms. Although some patients have found they can tolerate Thayers Slippery Elm Throat Lozenges and Ricola Natural Herb Cough Drops. Look in health food stores if these cough treatments are not found in local drug stores. Always try a new cough drop for only a few seconds. Often a cough drop is not as irritating and still helpful if it isn't finished.

Some research has shown honey to be more effective than over-the-counter cough syrup. Manuka honey is usually considered the most healing variety and can be found in health food stores.

IC/BPS patients should be cautious when trying prescription expectorants. The expectorant Humibid has been known to set off IC/BPS flare-ups, even when a very small amount is used. The generic form of Humibid, guaifenesin, is sometimes prescribed as a treatment for FMS. FMS patients with an irritable bladder may want to avoid this expectorant.

Certain herbal teas can help to soothe mucous membranes and loosen mucous. However, many of these herbal teas can also irritate the bladder. Safer alternatives include weak tea made from a little dried dill weed or parsley. These herbs are good for coughs and respiratory problems. Dried sage tea can be used to soothe sore throats. Sage tea can also be used as a gargle. White Sage and Wild Mint Tea (available at Isabella) makes a great gargle because white sage is an anti-inflammatory and antibacterial herb. The tea is also used for prostate health. It's best to make it very weak when first trying. Slippery elm and licorice root teas are both very soothing; however, licorice root is strong and not always tolerated by bladder-sensitive patients. Neem leaf tea also soothes throats and has strong antimicrobial properties. All teas should be tried using only one quick dunk of a tea bag or tea ball into a boiling cup of water.

For general aches and pains that come with the flu try plain (weak) chamomile tea. Chamomile is a great relaxant. For prevention of colds and infections try weak tea made of dried thyme. Thyme is also beneficial when used in cooked food. Both garlic (if tolerated) and mushrooms, especially shitake mushrooms, should be eaten regularly to prevent colds, flu, and respiratory infections.

Treating Migraine Headaches

Migraines, like IC/BPS, can be treated with antidepressants and drugs such as hydroxyzine. Other medications such as muscle relaxants and anti-inflammatories may affect the bladder. Drugs that contain a blood vessel constrictor, a sedative, or acetaminophen may create bladder pain and frequency.

Women are more prone to migraines and some experts believe that this is due to the fluctuation in estrogen levels, especially during perimenopause. One recent study showed that two-thirds of women with migraines, who have gone through natural menopause, find improvement. But on the other hand, women who have hysterectomies typically find that their migraines worsen. There seems to be a similar pattern with female IC/BPS patients. Many IC/BPS patients experience a flare-up of bladder symptoms right after a hysterectomy. Just as many find improvement in their IC/BPS after natural menopause.

Prevention of migraine headaches includes following a diet for IC/BPS patients and the avoidance of foods that contain monosodium glutamate, hot breads, hot raised coffee cakes, hot donuts (cold breads, cakes, and donuts are better), processed meats, and aged foods. For a more complete migraine diet list refer to neurologist David Buchholz's book, *Heal Your Headache*. Other triggers for migraines include fatigue, stress, bright lights, noise, missing meals, hormonal changes, birth control pills, progesterone, and fumes from perfume, paint, pesticides, and other toxic products. Preventive measures, such as diet, acupuncture, and trigger point therapy may be the best ways to treat migraine headaches.

Rubbing a little peppermint oil on your temples can help to ease a tension headache. People who suffer with chronic tension headaches should be checked for TMJD.

Anti-Inflammatory Medications

Anti-inflammatory medications are sometimes used to treat IC/BPS, but often over-the-counter and prescription anti-inflammatory oral medications, intended for the treatment of other conditions, may cause burning in the bladder and stomach upset. Reactions are very individual, but IC/BPS patients may want to avoid over-the-counter NSAIDs that contain caffeine and other irritating ingredients.

Cox-2 inhibitors such as Celebrex are used as anti-inflammatory pain relievers for arthritis. They are known for their many side effects including straining to urinate and painful urination. IC/BPS patients should if possible avoid Cox-2 inhibitors. Networking and connecting with other IC/BPS patients with similar conditions can be helpful.

Diet Medications and Stimulants

Because IC/BPS patients must often take medications, such as antidepressants and antihistamines, they gain weight that is hard to lose. Nevertheless, patients should never skip meals or consider taking a diet medication. Diet medications may not only trigger bladder symptoms, they can also affect patients who are chemically sensitive. Dieting to lose weight should be a slow process combined with bladder-friendly exercise and good nutrition. Skipping meals or starvation diets can worsen bladder symptoms. (Toxins are stored in fat cells and are mobilized when dieting.)

IC/BPS patients should try sensible dieting combined with exercise and physician supervision. Patients should be tested for allergies. Foods that act as allergens can also cause weight gain due to toxic build-up.

Perhaps, patients who would like to lose weight, or maintain a healthy weight, should add flaxseed to their diets. Flaxseed is believed to speed up metabolism and burn fat.

Pain Medications

Relieving any type of pain seems to be a challenge for IC/BPS patients. Pain medications can contain caffeine and other ingredients which irritate the bladder and stomach. Muscle relaxants prescribed to relieve other muscles in the body (not the smooth muscle of the bladder) may cause bladder pain and make it difficult for IC/BPS patients to fully urinate. Because many medications can adversely affect neurotransmitter levels and bodily functions in IC/BPS patients, pain prevention should be used instead as much as possible. *See Coping with General Conditions, Routine Exams, and Procedures without the Drugs and Fillers that Might Trigger IC/BPS Pain in this chapter.*

Dealing with Serious Chronic Conditions

When other conditions are serious, they can be hard to treat without disturbing the bladder. Thyroid disease, vitamin deficiencies, chronic heart conditions, high cholesterol, and other serious conditions and life-threatening illnesses require treatments and medications that can interfere with bladder maintenance in IC/BPS patients. Some patients would rather avoid a diagnosis or treatment of a serious condition because they are naturally afraid of an adverse reaction in their bladders. They may not take painful signs seriously, and may back away from doctors and new treatments because they were not helped in the past. IC/BPS patients may unconsciously choose to compromise their physical health to avoid physical pain, judgment, and dismissal. Chronic pain patients often become used to feeling lousy or being told that their various aches and pains are probably nothing, or just part of the disease, so they end up dismissing their symptoms. Dismissing symptoms can be dangerous to IC/BPS patients, especially as they grow older, because they may not take the aging process into account. Because IC/BPS patients become wary, they sometimes risk overlooking a serious condition.

When a new medication is necessary, you may need to experiment. However, with so many patients sharing the same overlapping conditions, you may be able to avoid "trial by error." For a wealth of patient information about medications and procedures refer to the IC Network. *See Resources.*

Colonoscopy Preparation Medicines

The colon must be cleared for the colonoscopy in order to view the surface of the large intestine (colon). Cleaning out the colon can be done in different ways and many patients seem to do just fine with the prep medications. But unfortunately there are patients who have experienced bladder symptoms such as burning or pelvic floor pain soon after trying prep medications. This may be due to the high sodium content and/or the dyes in the drinks. Prep medications are available in tablets and flavored liquids. A plain liquid drink is also available, which may be more desirable for patients who might react to the lemon-lime, cherry, and orange flavoring. Sometimes patients must take tablets along with liquid preparation, or additional fluids and laxatives depending on the type of preparation. An anti-nausea medication may be used to make the drink go through the body faster. (Patients who can tolerate Gatorade say that it helps with dehydration and electrolyte balance. Patients who cannot tolerate Gatorade can try coconut water, which is filled with electrolytes.)

When a patient cannot tolerate the preparation medications, they may consider having a colonic, which is like a powerful enema. However, it can be difficult to find a clinic that offers this procedure and some patients might be afraid that the procedure will trigger a bladder flare-up. But colonics are often bladder-friendly for patients. Most gastroenterologists will be open to this alternative just as long as their patients are clean for the colonoscopy. Patients with constipation IBS may also have to take a laxative such as Ducolax to clean the colon. If a patient is not entirely cleaned out, the doctor can use a strong enema before the procedure.

IC/BPS patients usually do well with the colonoscopy procedure, as well as the sedative that must be administered before the procedure. The colonoscopy takes about 30 to 60 minutes. During the colonoscopy the doctor may detect and remove polyps. This will not cause pain when the sedative wears off. If the polyps are the pre-cancerous type, a patient may have to have a repeat colonoscopy in a couple of years. It is crucial for IC/BPS patients to undergo a colonoscopy in order to avoid the risks of colon cancer. Colon cancer is not only very serious, it can require chemotherapy drugs and radiation, which can be very hard on the IC/BPS bladder.

B-12 Supplementation

IC/BPS patients should probably have their vitamin B-12 levels tested. Vitamin B-12 deficiency is fairly common, especially in vegetarians (B-12 is only found in animal sources), the elderly, people on long-term acid-suppressing drugs, and sometimes people with autoimmune disorders. Symptoms of this deficiency include: anemia, and/or nerve damage, insomnia, memory problems, and depression. Although B-12 deficiency can now be treated with a high-dose prescription oral medication or nasal spray, IC/BPS patients may do best with the old-fashioned injections. (B-12 is usually better tolerated than the other B vitamins.) Unfortunately, some patients diagnosed with pernicious anemia often have to fight for insurance coverage of their injections. Some insurance companies would rather cover oral medications.

Patients with borderline deficiency may have to convince their doctors that they need monthly injections.

Thyroid Disease

Hypothyroidism (underactive thyroid) is common in both fibromyalgia (FMS) and IC/BPS patients and is not reserved for older patients. Symptoms of hypothyroidism are discussed in Chapter One. Most doctors like to treat patients with Synthroid and Levoxyl, but these synthetic brands of thyroid can sometimes trigger bladder symptoms and anxiety in IC/BPS patients. If patients find they cannot tolerate the synthetic thyroid drugs, they can ask for natural Armour thyroid, which is made from pig thyroid. There are arguments pro and con for natural thyroid and a doctor will most probably prefer to prescribe a synthetic brand because it's easier to regulate. Although patients often do best with prescription natural thyroid, the different dosages may vary in filler content.

Some IC/BPS patients find that they must build their thyroid levels slowly and others, who must cut back on their dosage, should also do so slowly. Since thyroid levels can fluctuate, patients may need frequent testing. If patients' prescriptions are switched from a non-generic brand of thyroid medication to a generic medication, they will also need to be tested to determine levels.

There are some supplements and antidepressants that have an effect on the thyroid. According to *Graedons' People's Pharmacy,* "minerals such as calcium and iron affect absorption of Synthroid and Levoxyl." (Calcium will also interfere with the absorption of natural thyroid.) Antidepressants, such as Prozac and Effexor, have also been known to disrupt normal thyroid functioning. *For more information patients can order a* Guide to Thyroid Hormones. *See Resources.*

IC/BPS and FMS patients with borderline levels of thyroid may experience symptoms that need treatment, but not every doctor understands this. Hopefully, most doctors are aware that patients with hypothyroidism should be tested for vitamin D deficiency. This deficiency is very common in people with thyroid problems. *See Medications for the Reversal of Osteoporosis in this chapter for more information on vitamin D.*

Patients may want to try other natural thyroid medications, such as Nature-Throid or the Canadian brand Efra. Fillers in thyroid medication, such as cellulose, can vary and some brands are friendlier to the stomach.

Blood Pressure Medications

The best medicine for high blood pressure (hypertension) is prevention with lifestyle modifications, such as regular exercise and relaxation techniques, as well as a healthy diet that includes onions, garlic, sweet potatoes, Swiss chard, salmon, tuna, herring, anchovies, extra-virgin olive oil, beans, whole grains, blueberries, and blackberries (when tolerated). Some spices are also beneficial. Turmeric, an ingredient used in curry that appears to be bladder-safe for many patients, basil, thyme, and rosemary are all heart healthy. Onions (and some IC/BPS supplements mentioned in Chapter One) contain quercetin, which is thought to lower blood pressure. Slightly cooked garlic eaten on a daily basis may be very effective in reducing blood pressure. So is bladder-friendly food high in potassium. Both sweet potatoes and Swiss chard offer adequate amounts of potassium. Fish oil will also lower blood pressure, but some IC/BPS patients cannot tolerate fish oil. Instead, patients can add the oily fish mentioned above to their diets.

Cutting back on salt intake plays a role in lowering blood pressure. So does switching from conventional salt to a good quality rock salt because less is needed and rock salt offers more trace minerals than regular salt. The salty seaweed Dulse is packed with vitamins and minerals and, used sparingly, can replace table salt. Nori seaweed is another option to flavor food. Patients with high blood pressure should also consider The Dash Diet to lower their sodium intake.

Medications taken to treat high blood pressure can trigger IC/BPS symptoms. Patients with stage 1 hypertension are typically prescribed diuretics, which may increase frequency and possibly contain other irritating ingredients. Patients with hypertension that is higher than stage 1 usually must add another medication to relax or widen the blood vessels. Two such medications have actually been used to treat IC/BPS symptoms: calcium channel blockers, which inhibit smooth muscle contraction, and alpha blockers, which block certain hormones. Of course, these are not standard treatments for IC/BPS patients.

Because blood pressure medications often trigger bladder symptoms, patients might want to network with other IC/BPS patients to find the most bladder-safe medication. Some patients have found that older medications, such as Apresoline (hydralazine), don't have such an effect on their bladders. Another drug, which is newer, called Zestril (lisinopril), has also been tolerated by some patients, but it can cause coughing. Of course, every patient is individual. Since many of the medications for hypertension may trigger IC/BPS symptoms, patients need to use prevention by following a healthy diet, getting enough exercise, as well as quality sleep, to prevent this serious condition. *Patients should also refer to Dr. Andrew Weil's Guide to Heart Health.*

Some patients may experience "white coat" hypertension. This occurs when a patient is nervous or fearful about seeing the doctor and/or having the exam, which understandably may be the case with IC/BPS patients. Most patients have been through bad experiences with doctors and procedures.

Cholesterol-Lowering Medications

Statins, which are medications given to reduce cholesterol, can cause muscle cramps, enhancing the pain of fibromyalgia (FMS), and perhaps that of IC/BPS too. According to a 2004 Fibromyalgia Network Drug Update article, "Cholesterol-Lowering Meds Cause Muscle Pain," statins can interfere with CoQ production. CoQ is a vital enzyme that is required for muscle function. It is known that the commonly prescribed statin Lipitor (atorvastatin) may present problems for FMS patients. But, the statin Crestor (rosuvastatin) may be better tolerated because it has the lowest side effects of the statins. Another possible option for lowering cholesterol is Zetia (ezetimibe), which is a newer drug that works by minimizing the intestinal absorption of cholesterol. The FMS Network suggested that a combination of the lowest dose of both Zetia and Crestor may work well to lower cholesterol and have the least side effects. However, this does not necessarily mean that these drugs are bladder-safe.

Once again, a healthy lifestyle is the key to avoiding unhealthy cholesterol levels and irritating medications (although some people unfortunately inherit this condition). Eating the foods that were mentioned previously in "Blood Pressure Medications," eliminating bad fats and adding healthy fats to your diet can help to lower bad cholesterol. Good fats, such as Omega 3 fatty acids, are found in flax seeds, walnuts, nut butters like walnut, almond, and cashew, and oily fish (fish must be consumed twice, if not more, a week). A handful of pistachio nuts can help to lower bad cholesterol which is called LDL, and ground flax seed has many benefits, including reducing inflammation in the body and lowering LDL. Flax seed is actually more beneficial than flax seed oil, which is good news for IC/BPS patients who cannot tolerate supplemental oils. However, dietary oils like extra-virgin olive oil and canola oil are beneficial and easily added to patients' diets. Patients may also benefit from foods enriched with Omega 3.

People with high cholesterol should routinely exercise and practice relaxation. Emotional stress is known to raise cholesterol levels.

Flax seed must be ground to obtain its benefits. A small coffee grinder can be used. The ground seed may be refrigerated up to a week. For more information on high blood pressure, high cholesterol, and general heart health refer to Dr. Andrew Weil's Guide to Heart Health. *See Resources.*

Medications for the Reversal of Osteoporosis

There are IC/BPS patients who can tolerate these medications, but there are also many who experience bladder symptoms and other side effects when they try the various treatments for osteoporosis. Therefore, it's essential that both younger and older IC/BPS patients understand the importance of preventing osteoporosis. Every patient should consider the consequences of this po-tential condition, no matter their age or gender. Patients who have been on steroid therapy or female patients who have had their menses medically ceased should undergo a bone density scan.

Depending on your medical history and the medical history of your family members, you may want to get a little daily sunshine. Although controversial (there is quite a big vitamin-D debate go-ing on in the medical field), if there is adequate sunshine where you live, trying to sensibly get a little sun on your arms and the top of your head, as well as your back, for about 10 minutes on most days will produce vitamin D in your body. Needless to say, it's important to protect the gentle skin on your face and chest. Before exposing yourself to the sun get your doctor's blessing. Skin cancer can be very serious.

If you can tolerate vitamin D supplements, you are probably lucky and you should take them (calcium absorption is depen-dent on vitamin D). If you cannot take supplements, see if you can tolerate fish oil. There are a couple of different fish oils to choose from, like herring and marine oils. (As mentioned earlier supplemental oils can be irritating to some patients' bladders.) If you're a patient who cannot tolerate vitamin D supplements or fish oil, you can add egg yolks, milk, liver, and oily fish to your diet. You can also try drinks that are enriched with vitamin D, such as Rice Dream, Coconut Dream, and Almond Breeze. Rice Dream and Coconut Dream may be better tolerated because Al-mond Breeze contains some minerals that may bother the IC/BPS bladder. Some patients believe that the irritant in almond milk is the additive carrageenan.

One study has shown that low blood levels of vitamin D can lead to a heart attack or a stroke.

Besides absorption from the sun and diet, people can actu-ally raise their levels of vitamin D with medical phototherapy. Not every doctor knows or agrees with this, but phototherapy has been proven to raise vitamin D levels. Even so, insurance companies won't cover phototherapy for this purpose. However, there is another way to raise vitamin D levels, which is visiting a tanning salon three times a week. This prescription for vitamin D, of course, is not considered as safe as medical phototherapy.

When women reach the age of 50, they become candidates for a bone density scan to detect osteopenia (the condition that can lead to osteoporosis) or osteoporosis. If osteoporosis is detected, a patient is typically prescribed bisphosphonates to maintain bone density and reverse bone loss. Fosamax (alendronate sodium), Boniva (ibandronate sodium) and Actonel (risedronate sodium) are all oral biophosphonates prescribed for osteoporosis. Oral bisphosphonates cannot be cut, but Boniva can be delivered in an injection. Determining if a Boniva injection is tolerable is a little difficult, but a nurse or doctor can administer a small amount of the injection, just enough for only one week. So, if the drug isn't bladder-friendly, you will not have to endure 3 months of symptoms. Of course, it takes an understanding doctor who realizes that the small dose is an experiment and that the patient knows it is not therapeutic.

Reclast (zoledronic acid) is another bisphosphonate that can be taken orally or given in an intravenous injection. Oral Reclast cannot be cut and the injection is very long lasting. Again, experimenting with a very small amount of the injection is essential before putting such a long-acting drug into your body. Since Reclast has an effect on estrogen receptors in the body, it may have an adverse effect on the bladder. Aside from bladder symptoms patients may experience other side effects with bisphosphonates, such as digestive problems and pain in their joints and muscles that may occur mostly in their arms and legs. Occasionally, medications that list leg pain as a possible side effect can also affect the pelvic floor and the bladder. The legs attach to the boney part of the pelvis and the muscles of the hips are part of the pelvic muscles.

Other classes of osteoporosis medication include the drugs Forteo (teriparatide) and Fortical (calcitonin, salmon). Forteo is a synthetic version of the parathyroid hormone, which regulates calcium and phosphates in your bones. This drug is reserved for severe osteoporosis in both women and men, and is given in daily injections. Not much is known about Forteo because it is fairly new, but it has been known to cause IC/BPS symptoms in some patients. Fortical is a nose spray made of a synthetic version of salmon calcitonin. It works with the parathyroid to regulate calcium levels. Fortical is very hard on the nasal passages and may cause urinary burning and pain in some people. A newer medication called Prolia (denosumab) also reverses osteoporosis but is delivered in a twice yearly injection and there are many side effects. Long lasting drugs are usually too risky for IC/BPS patients. Medications to reverse bone loss are still new to medicine and although they may be very helpful, some patients may need to turn to alternative methods to prevent and reverse bone loss.

Biosil (orthosilicic acid) is an oral supplement taken to promote the growth and development of the skin, hair, nails, and bones. It contains silicon which is a natural essential trace element in the body. Biosil offers many other benefits, but it appears to work best on facilitating bone mineralization. Can IC/BPS patients tolerate this supplement? The answer may be the same as it always is—tolerance is individual.

Vivian Goldschmidt, founder of Save Our Bones and graduate of New York University with a Master's degree in Nutritional Sciences and Biochemistry, has her own theory on bone health. Goldschmidt believes that medications to treat osteoporosis are toxic and actually compromise bone composition. In her experience the key to preventing, stopping, and reversing bone loss is keeping an alkaline environment in the body tissues. This can be achieved with a diet high in alkaline and low in acidity. Otherwise, if body tissues are acid, calcium and other minerals are used to neutralize the acidity depleting our bones of calcium. Goldschmidt lists alkalizing and acidifying foods and how to combine them in her book, *The Bone Health Revolution*. Although she makes a very good point, most doctors would probably disagree with Goldschmidt's theory, at least for now.

Foods That Help Prevent Toxic Build-up

We've all seen the TV commercials that advertise prescription drugs and we've probably noticed how they often advise people to have liver function tests before trying their drugs. This is because drugs are generally tough on the liver, which is the organ responsible for filtering toxins in the body. IC/BPS patients who must take drugs can easily add cleansing foods to their diets. The following foods will help to cleanse the liver and help to keep the body's tissue healthy:

- Cabbage
- Garlic
- Greens—kale, spinach, collard, turnip and mustard greens, broccoli, arugula, and bok choy
- Asparagus
- Acorn squash
- Avocados (if tolerated)
- Artichokes
- Beets
- Watermelon (if tolerated)
- Whole Grains

Coffee enemas can be used when liver enzymes are elevated, but this cleansing treatment should be discussed with a doctor.

Resources

Dr. Ann McCampbell
(505) 466-3622 • DrAnnMcC@gmail.com

Books

Dr. Andrew Weil's Guide to Heart Health
www.drweil.com

A Guide to Thyroid Hormones, Graedons' People's Pharmacy
www.peoplespharmacy.com

Products

The Vermont Country Store
www.vermontcountrystore.com • (800) 547-7849

Isabella
www.IsabellaCatalog.com
(800) 777-5205 (orders) • (888) 481-6745 (questions)

Baar Products
www.baar.com• (800) 269-2502

Lowell Foods
www.LowellInternationalFoods.com
(Cucumbers in Brine are also available at Amazon.)

Tomorrow's World
www.tomorrowsworld.com • (800) 229-7571

Gaiam
www.gaiam.com• (877) 989-6321

Earth's Botanical Harvest
www.aminoman.net • (800) 952-7921

Chapter Six

UNDERSTANDING CHEMICAL SENSITIVITIES AND ENVIRONMENTAL ILLNESS

Chemicals and toxins are all around us and can have an impact on people with a dysfunctional immune system (people who cannot properly detoxify chemicals). Chemicals can also be responsible for a dysfunctional immune system. A number of IC/BPS patients experience sensitivity to fragrances and scented products, and occasionally experience bladder symptoms when they are exposed to gasoline fumes, paints, pesticides, and certain chemicals. Some IC/BPS patients believe that they suffered with sensitivity before they had IC/BPS. Patients with mitral valve prolapse (MVP), hypothyroidism, and chronic fatigue syndrome (CFS) appear to be more sensitive to chemicals, and some research has shown a connection between chemical sensitivity and severe fibromyalgia (FMS).

This chapter will cover the chemical related illness called multiple chemical sensitivity (MCS). Although having IC/BPS does not mean that one is, or will become chemically sensitive, a spectrum of sensitivities and suggestions will be covered to meet the needs of a varied audience. Also, the following chapter is not limited strictly to the MCS patient, but is instead geared to bring attention to the various environmental factors that may have an impact on some IC/BPS patients. Neither is the information in this chapter intended as medical advice nor is it an endorsement of products and services. Many facts and suggestions come from hand-outs shared at support groups, and great effort has been made to give credit; however, in some cases proper credit might have been inadvertently omitted.

Multiple Chemical Sensitivity

MCS is defined as a chronic condition which is marked by a greatly increased sensitivity to multiple chemicals and other irritating substances. At least 30 percent of the American population experiences some symptoms of MCS. Symptoms range from mild to severe. Severe reactions to low levels of common chemicals can be serious, and sometimes life threatening.

MCS is also referred to as: environmental illness, sick building syndrome, chemical injury, and quite accurately, twentieth-century disease. But, because the condition does not fit traditional beliefs of the mechanisms of disease, most doctors don't know how to explain it. This is the reason why the American Medical Association (AMA) and so many traditional doctors, including some occupational health physicians, believe MCS to be psychosomatic, not organic. Even so, the Americans with Disabilities Act recognizes MCS as a disability and there is a specific branch of medicine called clinical ecology (also known as environmental medicine).

MCS Is Not a New Condition

This condition has been on the rise since the end of World War II (over 60 years ago) when manufacturers started using pesticides left over from the War. From that time, the production of organic chemicals, plastics, and synthetic fibers has rapidly increased. We now live in a very toxic world and, although not everyone develops MCS, many people get cancer and other conditions from everyday products.

Causes of MCS

Individuals initially become sensitized to chemicals, odors, fumes, and substances after repeated low-level exposure to chemicals, after an acute, high-level exposure to one chemical substance, or after exposure to mold. MCS becomes chronic when sensitivity increases and very low levels of scents and odors affect the body and the behavioral response to these substances. Some IC/BPS patients believe that chemicals have played a role in the development of their IC/BPS. The limbic system, which is affected by the pain and responsible for the emotions connected to IC/BPS, also regulates the sense of smell. Jay Gottfried, assistant professor of neurology at Northwestern University's Feinberg School of Medicine, explains that the average person detects thousands of scents subliminally even though he or she may only be aware of a few scents. He backs the studies that have shown that these undetected low levels of scents affect behavior. The patient with MCS detects most all scents and chemicals immediately, which has a profound and devastating effect.

Physical Symptoms of MCS

The body is exposed to toxins and allergens through substances that are inhaled, touched, eaten, applied in, or on the body. The most common symptoms of MCS are experienced in the sinuses, respiratory system, and central nervous system. Many of the reactions to chemicals are similar to the symptoms of allergies:

- headaches, including migraines and sinus pain
- hacking coughs
- bronchitis
- dizziness
- tremors
- swelling of the lips, tongue, and eyes
- allergic conjunctivitis
- dermatitis
- fatigue
- cardiac symptoms, such as palpitations and irregular heart beats
- muscle and joint pain
- numbness
- flu-like symptoms and colds

- low-grade fever
- depression

Reactions can cause:
- genitourinary problems
- gastrointestinal distress
- hyper-reactive behavior
- confusion
- difficulty with concentration
- short-term memory loss
- hyperactivity in children
- learning disabilities in children

Recognizing that children are increasingly suffering with asthma and other symptoms of chemical sensitivity, many cities and states are making non-toxic cleaning products mandatory in schools. Certain cities have banned pesticide use in playgrounds and public parks.

The neurotoxic effects of chemicals can impair functioning. Exposure to certain chemicals, pesticides, and industrial chemicals can lead to sensitization of the nerve in the nose, neurogenic inflammation, neurological injury, liver damage, and cancer (including bladder cancer). Certain pesticides and detergents contain estrogen-like substances (molecular structures that are similar to the body's own hormones). These chemicals go to the endocrine system where they mimic the effects of estrogen and contribute to an excess of estrogen and an imbalance of hormones in the body. Other chemicals, such as petrochemicals (petroleum products), penetrate the fatty tissue of the body. Although scientists have identified the potentially toxic effects of chemicals, there is still more that they must learn.

When continuously exposed to high levels of certain chemicals, anyone can be affected.

Treatment for MCS

Because MCS is best treated and prevented with avoidance, it's necessary to read as much as possible in order to make needed lifestyle changes. There are many books that address this illness. Support groups are also helpful and usually have current information. *To find a local support group contact the Human Ecology Action League (HEAL) listed in Resources.*

Environmental consultants, who are knowledgeable about chemical sensitivity, are often necessary when buying a new home, remodeling, building, or trying to identify sources of problems in the home and workspace. *To find a consultant contact other MCS patients, environmental or occupational physicians, environmental health departments at local universities, or refer to Resources.* Although environmental consultants are often listed online and sometimes in the yellow pages, it's necessary to find a consultant who is familiar with MCS.

Doctors who specialize in environmental illness are referred to as "environmental physicians" or "occupational physicians." Many of these specialists treat patients with overactive immune dysfunction and degenerative diseases such as systemic lupus, rheumatoid arthritis, and chronic fatigue syndrome (CFS). These physicians are familiar with the limitations of various illnesses, and should respect the IC/BPS patient's particularly sensitive needs. They should also be able to help hospitalized patients to avoid air pollution in the hospital room, as well as find safe medical supplies and equipment. One such physician is Ann McCampbell, M.D. *See Resources in Chapter Five.*

Patients with MCS who are physically able are sometimes advised to exercise and create a sweat in order to mobilize and excrete the toxins stored in the body's fat. A sauna, especially after exercise, to further encourage the release of toxins may also be recommended. This prescription might not be good advice for most IC/BPS patients, especially those on dehydrating medications.

Some alternative physicians gear their treatment to correct an imbalance of the endocrine, neurological, and immune systems. These physicians may prescribe detoxification, as well as systemic enzymes, minerals, and vitamins to repair biochemical damage. Alternative doctors may also test for magnesium deficiency. A few studies have shown that correcting a magnesium deficiency in a chemically sensitive person improves her or his MCS symptoms. Balanced zinc levels are also very important because zinc helps systemic enzymes to function and enzymes modulate the immune system. More studies are needed to really understand the role of supplements in improving the symptoms of MCS in patients.

Sensitive IC/BPS patients may want to try children's minerals and enzymes if they cannot tolerate the adult strength supplements, but the vitamins suggested for MCS patients are often in mega doses. Elimination of certain foods can sometimes be a helpful alternative to supplements. A number of IC/BPS patients have found that eliminating gluten (especially wheat), as well as dairy, yeast, and processed foods, which can contain chemicals and possibly irradiated ingredients, improves their tolerance to chemical exposure, therefore reducing their reactions. *See Chapter Two.*

Supplements and liquids taken for detoxification are usually not bladder-safe for IC/BPS patients. Treatments that chelate (attach to a toxin to draw it out of the body) toxins in order to cleanse the body can be very harmful if not done slowly under close supervision. Such treatments should probably be avoided by IC/BPS patients because the toxins have to pass through the bladder. IC/BPS patients may also have problems with MCS testing and techniques such as Enzyme Potentiated Desensitization (EPD). This technique desensitizes patients to their allergies with immunotherapy, using small doses of allergens. A strict regime and special diet must be followed. EPD may not be advisable for IC/BPS patients.

The IC/BPS patient's treatment for MCS should include the least intrusive methods: the avoidance of irritating chemicals, eating healthy foods, which may include giving up the culprit foods mentioned earlier, and practicing the right type of exercise. Patients must only exercise in a clean air environment, because air intake, both good and bad, is increased during exercise. If swimming is a choice, patients should find a pool treated by non-chlorinated methods. Salt water pools may be tolerable and are a healthy option. Local pool companies usually have information on alternative disinfectants; however, some alternatives (such as bromine) may be irritating. *For more information contact the American Environmental Health Foundation, Inc. (AEHF). Refer to Resources.*

Patients with MCS and IC/BPS should avoid any form of fasting. Fasting and regular dieting release toxins that are stored in body fat. If patients must diet for weight loss, it should be a slow process combined with gentle exercise under a doctor's supervision.

Can a Traditional Allergist Help a Patient with MCS?

Most allergists specialize in patients who suffer with traditional allergies and test positive for allergies. Patients who suffer with environmental illness are *sensitive* but not necessarily *allergic*. Even though many MCS patients react to molds and pollens after they become chemically sensitive, they may not test positive for allergies with standard allergy testing.

Many traditional allergists still believe that the symptoms of MCS are in a patient's head, or not of an *organic* cause. This idea is sometimes further supported by a patient's behavioral reaction to chemicals and irritants. Reactions to chemicals and irritants can be quite severe, eccentric, and very misunderstood. The MCS patient may appear to health-care professionals as a victim of trauma or abuse, when in actuality, they may be susceptible to chemical reactions because of a genetic weakness. (The sense of smell is regulated by the limbic system, which involves pain processing and emotional responses.) This weakness often requires strong life control, and the need to act quickly and urgently when symptoms are triggered. Like IC/BPS, there is not much understood about this illness, probably less than IC/BPS. But the MCS patient knows all too well that she or he is the canary or guinea pig for the rest of the population.

Taking Control of Your Environment

If you believe that you experience MCS, or would like to improve your environment to prevent it, begin by replacing personal-care products that you feel may be irritating. Be sure to read labels carefully before trying new products and remember that no one product or process is assumed safe for everyone with chemical sensitivity.

Personal-Care Products

Personal-care products are used on or in your body. They include lotions, cosmetics, nail polish and remover, shampoos and conditioners, gels, hair sprays and hair dyes, perfumes and after shaves, deodorants and soaps, toothpaste and mouthwash. Most scented products today are petrochemical neurotoxins. Ninety-five percent of the chemicals in fragrances are synthetic compounds derived from petroleum. The contents of these fragrances have been found to be capable of causing cancer, birth defects, central nervous system disorders, and allergic reactions, such as eczema and the symptoms of MSC. These findings are not new. They were reported in 1986 by the Committee on Science and Technology, U.S. House of Representatives.

Cosmetic additives are another serious concern because their synthetic chemicals can be potentially toxic to the liver, kidneys, and endocrine system. In the book *Exposed*, investigative reporter Mark Shapiro reveals that the average American adult is exposed to more than one hundred distinct chemicals from personal-care products every day, and that women are especially exposed through the make-up and beauty products they use. Because of these findings the European Union's Cosmetics Directive has banned all chemicals determined as carcinogens, mutagens, or reproductive toxins from cosmetics sold in Europe. Several other countries have followed their lead, but as of yet, the United States has not. This is not to say that there isn't concern. There are concerned senators and representatives who are fighting for stricter consumer safety regulations.

A study by the University of Southern California School of Medicine showed that women using hair dyes at least once a month for a year are twice as likely to develop bladder cancer than women who do not use hair dye.

It takes time and money to replace irritating products with suitable ones. Even if your search begins in a health food store, you will probably have to sift through highly scented products (even organic products) and read labels if you wish to avoid silicone compounds and other questionable ingredients. Most cosmetics, shampoos, and hair products contain silicone additives. These additives may be listed as dimethicone, simethicone, and cyclomethicone. Silicone may be harmful to some people. Adverse reactions can cause FMS symptoms, including skin rashes. Many of the less expensive, old fashioned cosmetics and creams do not contain silicone. Companies specializing in natural and organic products usually carry some silicone-free products. Be sure to double check every product, because ingredients may change.

When possible, unscrew the tops of personal-care products to take a sniff test before buying, but never hold the products too close to your nose.

The comfort of each individual varies and naturally will dictate what should or should not be used. However, it's important to be aware that products labeled *hypoallergenic* do not necessarily protect a person with MCS, and products labeled *unscented* may still contain chemicals and/or masking fragrances. The term *natural* does not necessarily mean *organic,* and organic personal-care products do not have to fit the labeling standards of the National Organic Standards Act. Products can be labeled *organic* if they contain just one ingredient grown in accordance with the guidelines. Although USDA-certified organic cosmetics follow the same rules as USDA-certified organic food, the Consumers Union Eco Labels center believes that many of the products labeled "certified-organic" also contain synthetic ingredients. A third party, a trade group called the Natural Products Association (NPA), has been developed to enforce the term "natural." The NPA requires that 95 percent of the ingredients of a product be natural flora, fauna, or animal by-products (milk, honey, and beeswax) and that there will be no harm to animals. States like California and Minnesota have taken action. California has a Safe Cosmetics Act and Minnesota has banned the use of mercury in mascara, eyeliners and skin lightening creams.

According to the *Green Guide* the following cosmetic lines are the likeliest to adhere to the European Union standards, which are stricter than the standards of the United States:

- NVEY ECO
- PHYSICIANS FORMULA ORGANIC WEAR
- SUKI COLOR
- DR. HAUSCHKA

There are several other very good, synthetic-free cosmetic and personal-care companies, such as Vincenza Skin Actives, Real Purity, Aroma Bella, Lavera, Miessence, Hemp Organics, Earth's Beauty, and Biologika.

Of course, there are natural scents in safe cosmetics that may be unsuitable for people with MCS and some people without MCS. A study printed in the *British Journal of Dermatology* showed that popular natural ingredients such as tea tree oil, feverfew, lavender, and jasmine caused an allergic response or a sensitivity response in some of the participants in the study. Again, tolerance of scents is very individual, but patients can easily avoid toxins by referring to the *Green Guide's* "Dirty Dozen." The "Dirty Dozen" is a list of hazardous ingredients in personal-care products that can have serious health impacts:

- **Antibacterials**
- **Coal-tar colors** found in "FD&C" or "D&C" colors found in makeup and hair dye (FD&C Blue 1, FD&C Green 3, D&C Red 33, FD&C Yellow 5, FC&C Yellow 6)
- **Diethanolamine (DEA)** (found in shampoos) and its compounds and derivatives such as **triethanolamine (TEA),**

which can be contaminated with nitrosamines compounds which may cause cancer, especially if the product also contains **Bronopol**

- **1,4-Dioxane** (present in **sodium laureth sulfate (SLES)** and **sodium lauryl sulfate (SLS)** and other -eth ingredients)
- **Formaldehyde** found in eye shadows, mascaras, nail polish, and other cosmetics, and in a liquid state is labeled as **DMDM hydantoin, diazolidinyl urea, imidazolidinyl urea.** and **quaternium-15**
- **Fragrance** which contains phthalates found in deodorants, nail polishes (Today there are phthalate-free nail polishes, hair products, lotions, and, of course, fragrance.)
- **Hydroquinone,** a neurotoxin used in skin-lightening creams
- **Mercury** (allowed in a small amount) used as a preservative in eye-area cosmetics and **lead** (Lead acetate is found in hair dyes and make-up.)
- **Nanoparticles** are sometimes used medically to deliver drugs, but there is concern about their effects if they enter the bloodstream
- **Parabens**: methyl-, **propyl-**, ethyl-, butyl-, and isobutyl are common preservatives in cosmetics that mimic estrogen
- **Petroleum distillates** (such as petroleum jelly and mineral oil)
- **Phenylenediamine (PPD)** found in hair dyes and banned in Europe

Organic Color Systems offers ammonia-free, natural, organic, vegan, and cruelty-free hair products to hair stylists. These products do have a scent, but it is not a chemical smell.

Other toxic ingredients used in personal-care products:

- Dibutyl phthalate (DBP) a phthalate found in nail polishes and mascara
- Dimethyl phthalate (DMP) and diethyl phthalate (DEP) often hide behind the term "fragrance"

- Bronopol, or listed as 2-bromo-2-nitropropane-1,3-diol, can break down to produce formaldehyde
- Quaternary ammonium compounds such as Quaternium-15, which causes more complaints than any other preservative according to the American Academy of Dermatology
- Aluminum chlorohydrate used in antiperspirants
- Ammonia found in hair dyes and bleaches
- Peroxide used in hair coloring
- Polyethylene and polyethylene glycol (PEG ingredients) found in hair straighteners, antiperspirants, and baby-care products and can be contaminated with 1,4-dioxane
- Polysorbate compounds 60 and 80 used in lotions and creams and can become contaminated with the carcinogen 1,4-dioxane
- Polyvinylpyrrolidone (PVP) in hair products, especially hair sprays
- Propylene glycol found in mascara, lotions, creams, and other cosmetics
- Talc, a mineral found in many face and body powders, has a structure similar to that of asbestos, which has been linked to lung and ovarian cancers
- Toluene, a solvent found in some nail polishes, is a nervous-system toxin (California classifies conventional nail polish as hazardous waste. MCS patients usually feel the effects of toluene very quickly.)
- Triclosan, an antibacterial agent found in deodorants and other products, is linked to antibiotic-resistant disease

Mineral make-up may be a healthy choice for women because it doesn't promote bacteria and therefore doesn't need preservatives.

Because almost any product, including those that are labeled "certified organic," can affect you when you are sensitive, it's very important to be conservative when first trying something new. Always test your body with a small amount and be cautious when applying lotions to the buttocks and inner thigh area. Keep in mind that oils and lotions can travel, and lotions containing menthol and citrus can transfer from the hands to the toilet tissue and onto the urethra. (Hand sanitizers can also transfer to the urethra. Let hand sanitizers dry thoroughly before touching toilet tissue.) Shampoos containing strong fragrance and/or medication, such as dandruff shampoo, or a shampoo with natural tea tree oil, can come into contact with the urethra as well. It may be safer to shampoo in the sink rather than the shower when using strong shampoos.

> *Toilet tissue can contain dioxin, therefore patients may want to do a little research on the tissue they use.*

Bath oils, herbs, and bubble bath are other irritants that can affect the urethra and trigger IC/BPS symptoms. In place of these try adding baking soda or a little sea salt to your bath water. Avoid irritating chlorine by placing a water filter on your bathtub faucet. Eliminate chloroform gas, which affects the eyes, nose, and lungs, by placing a filter on your shower head. Systems to treat the whole home water supply are also available. *For information on water filters, call the American Environmental Health Foundation, Inc. (AEHF), National Ecological and Environmental Delivery Systems (N.E.E.D.S), or CWR Environmental Products. Refer to Resources.*

> *When showering in chlorinated water one absorbs more chlorine than drinking 8 glasses of chlorinated tap water.*

Sensitivities are highly individual. When making modifications and replacing products, begin with the products you use the most. Be sure to read all new product labels for ingredients and ask questions about everything. Always use your instincts. If you feel the slightest bit uncomfortable with a product, don't use it. Look for a Period After Opening (PAO) icon on products. This number logo displays how many months the product will be safe after opening. For instance, "5M" would mean five months. Displaying a PAO logo on products is mandatory on European products with a shelf life of thirty or more months. Although some companies have voluntarily followed the European lead, the logo is not yet required in the U.S.

The Food and Drug Administration (FDA) does not regulate cosmetics. To check the safety of a cosmetic, refer to safecosmetics.org and thecosmeticsdatabase.com. To find cosmetics without synthetics and strong fragrances refer to Allnaturalcosmetics.com, holisticbeauty.net, naturalorganicguide.com, and everyday-organics.com. Remember to ask about natural fragrances in products. To avoid phthalates in personal care products refer to nottoopretty.org.

Probably one of the most important personal care products that should be organic is deodorant. Conventional deodorants use synthetic chemicals to block odor and prevent sweating. Some of these chemicals have actually been found in breast tumors. There are several options for organic deodorants, including crystal deodorants (found at health food stores), and Tom's of Maine, which work fine for many people, but they don't always block odor. Those who need something stronger may want to try Green People No Scent Roll-On Deodorant, Lāfes Deodorant Spray (www.Lafes.com), Pit Powder Deodorant for women, or Pit Stop Powder Deodorant for men (these last two do have a scent). *Refer to Isabella in Chapter Five Resources.*

New Clothing

New clothing usually contains strong dyes, dry cleaning solution, masking fragrances, and sometimes fire retardant. Imported clothing may be treated with pesticides. Pure wool may be mothproofed. Even clothing and materials labeled natural or organic aren't always safe.

If you buy a piece of clothing that has a distinct odor or is chemically irritating, you can try adding a half-cup of baking soda or washing soda and a quarter cup of vinegar to your detergent before washing. If the odor is very strong, you may want to follow this cleaning recipe taken from a support group handout or refer to the book *Less Toxic Living*:

- Soak clothing in a bucket of cold water with about ½ cup of powdered milk (do not put powdered milk in the washing machine) for no more than 24 hours.
- Next wash with a tolerated soap.
- Soak clothing for another 24 hours in cold water with ½ cup each of baking soda and white vinegar.
- Rewash in a tolerated soap, and dry.

Wools and silks (not always the linings in clothes) can usually be hand washed in cold water with baking soda or a tolerated detergent, such as Free and Clear Seventh Generation or Ecos Free and Clear. Clothes should be hung to dry instead of using dryer heat because heat releases chemicals. Ironing releases chemicals in treated fabrics as well, so it's necessary to use proper ventilation. It's also important to avoid irons with Teflon surfaces and cookware coated with Teflon.

Synthetic clothing can cause itching and irritation, as well as MCS symptoms. MCS patients should eliminate clothing and sheets containing polyester or permanent-press, because they may also contain formaldehyde. Several clothes manufacturers offer natural fiber clothing labeled as "Certified Organic Cotton" or "Linen" and "Certified Organic" or "PuregrowWool," grown without synthetic pesticides and fertilizers. These companies include Patagonia, Eco Sport, Maggie's Functional Organics, Tomorrow's World, Way It Should Be, Earth Wear Organic Cotton Originals, Blue Canoe, and Nike Organics.

Like most clothes, shoes usually contain toxic chemicals, including benzene-based glues, soft plastics, dyes, and waterproofing sprays. Obviously, new shoes should be well aired-out before wearing. And, although there are now companies that make greener shoes, "green" does not necessarily make a product safe for MCS patients. It simply means that the product is not as harmful to people and the earth as a non-green product. However, companies like Adidas, New Balance, Nike, Puma, and Reebok have eliminated PVC and reduced VOCs in their shoes, which does help the MCS patient. According to the *The Green Guide*, women's handbags, beach bags, totes, and some luggage contain PVC vinyl liners, which release dioxins. The MSC person will usually be able to sense the strong odor instantly when they are near PVC vinyl products.

Dry cleaning is an obvious irritant, but there are now cleaners who use alternatives called *wet cleaning* or *CO2 cleaning* (which uses tension and steam), *green cleaning* or *organic cleaning* (which eliminate solvents called perchloroethylene, or perc). Some cleaners have switched their perc to perc-alternatives that use hydrocarbon solvents. Dry cleaners can use these solvents in their old perc machines and, even though they are considered healthier for the environment than perc, they probably should be avoided. Liquid silicone cleans very well, but may also present a problem for patients. The health effects have not yet been fully researched. *To find alternative dry cleaning, look up hangersdrycleaners.com and greenearthcleaning.com.* Some people avoid the dry cleaners by only wearing washable clothing.

> *Although there are no regulations on dry cleaners, federal law plans to phase out perc cleaners located in residential buildings by 2020. As it stands, perc cleaners are already limited in California. All clothes cleaned with perc should be aired out for at least three days before wearing.*

Using someone else's washing machine and dryer, or sharing washing machines and dryers with others (unless only unscented detergent and fabric softeners/sheets have been used in the appliances) can also present a problem. Conventional laundry detergents and fabric softeners contain heavy fragrance, which usually contains phthalates (hormone disruptors) to make the fragrance last longer. The fragrance lingers in the washing machine and dryer and will end up on your clothes even if you use your own unscented organic detergent. Chemical residue from dryer sheets also lingers on lint filters in dryers.

Bleaching clothes presents health problems, as well. Chlorine bleach can burn the respiratory tract, and burn the eyes and skin. Hydrogen peroxide can be used in place of ordinary bleach or chlorine-free bleach can be used. These can be found at health food stores and some grocery stores. Mindy Pennybacker, author of *Do One Green Thing,* uses the following recipe to whiten clothes:

- Presoak clothes in 2 tsp. washing soda mixed with 1 gallon water in a pan, or add ½ cup of washing soda to your wash load before starting.
- Add ½ cup of Borax or white vinegar in 1 gallon of water during the wash cycle, or lemon juice and water at the rinse cycle. (Always wear gloves.)
- Hang clothes in the sun after washing to whiten.

Cleaning up Your Home Environment

Indoor Air Quality

Your home is important. The better you take care of your needs at home, the better you can take care of your life and the people in it.

Many products sold to relieve allergies in the home are intended for people with traditional allergies and not intended for people with chemical sensitivity. Plastic and vinyl covers used to prevent dust mites can make those who are chemically sensitive ill. Instead, a barrier cloth can be used to cover furniture. Better yet, is to use organic bedding that naturally repels dust mites. Sheets and bedding used on conventional mattresses should be washed in hot water to control dust mites and their fecal matter.

Conventional brands of mattresses may contain many chemicals including pesticides, the fire retardant polybrominated diphenyl ethers (PBDE), bleach, stain and water resistant treatments. (Mattresses made with memory foam may contain even more toxins.) Plus, the amount of fire retardant used in mattresses has increased in the past several years. Because of this, chemical-free mattresses are becoming very popular, and although they are expensive, they are often necessary for sensitive people. Otherwise, a new chemically laden mattress will have to be aired-out for a few months to avoid breathing in strong odors while sleeping; but the mattress will still contain harmful chemicals that can cause sinus pain, breathing problems, and migraine headaches. In contrast, the natural materials used in organic mattresses include untreated cotton, wool (containing lanolin, a natural dust mite repellent), silk, pesticide-free flax, fresh natural rubber from the rubber tree, green tea, corn, petrochemical-free latex, and water-based polyurethane. Wool can be naturally treated with fire-retarding sea salt, but green mattresses containing pine should be avoided by people with MCS. The company LifeKind offers America's #1-Selling Organic Mattress, but there are many other companies that offer organic mattresses, such as Vivetique Sleep Systems. *For more information on removing toxins from your sleep environment refer to* Sleep Safe in a Toxic World *by Walter Bader.*

> *PBDEs are also released by crumbling foam in furniture. Two PBDEs have been banned in California.*

Organic bedding, sheets, pillows, bedspreads, and towels can be ordered from Gaiam Living, Cozy Pure (Tomorrow's World), and Lifekind. A natural alternative to a memory foam pillow is the Keetsa Tea Leaf pillow with no VOCs. *See Resources.* Vinyl shower curtains and liners should be replaced with shower curtains made of hemp, canvas, or linen (they need no liner but need to be washed often). If a liner is preferred, choose an Eco Shower Curtain Liner, which is made of chloride and odor free EVA (ethylene vinyl acetate). Or choose a liner made of PEVA (polyethylene vinyl acetate). Both EVA and PEVA do not contain phthalates, organotins, or vinyl chloride. They are sold at Ikea. com. Vita Futura offers healthy bathroom accessories, such as shower curtains and safety bath and shower mats. Gaiam Living, Cozy Pure, and Lifekind also carry healthy shower curtains.

> *Toxic dioxins are a by-product of PVC vinyl production, as well as chlorine bleaching. Clear plastic/vinyl shower curtains and liners contain PVC.*

Cleaning Products

Replacing your cleaning products can make life more comfortable instantly. Keeping the environment and air quality clean and free of toxic fumes, mold, mildew, and dust is vital to your health if you are sensitive. Begin changing your cleaning products by replacing chlorine bleach and products containing bleach. Stop using conventional dishwashing soap. Dishwashing soaps are not well regulated and their synthetic fragrances can contain phthalates (hormone disruptors), as well as many other chemicals. Stop using ammonia, commercial floor and furniture polishes, oven cleaners, waxes, and strippers. Avoid air fresheners and room deodorizers. These products usually make rooms smell better by desensitizing the olfactory nerve in the nose. This process backfires in people with MCS. Instead, they have terrible reactions to these chemicals, which are absolutely not healthy for anyone. Phthalates linger for months. Natural fragrances do not; they just evaporate. Scented candles are another concern, especially conventional synthetic and petroleum-based candles. Patients should only use natural beeswax candles and avoid all pine scented candles, cleaners, and disinfectants (even organic), as they are bad for people with MCS. Air can be cleaned naturally with a Salt Lamp (available at Isabella, *see Resources in Chapter Five*). Salt lamps emit negative-ions that refresh the air and recharge the body. Many people tout their negative ion machines because these machines help with health issues, such as sinus and breathing problems. *Refer to negative ion generators by Comtech Research.* Patients should always avoid ozone machines to clean air. Ozone is a chemical oxidant.

Again, instead of bleaching clothes with chlorine bleach, try hydrogen peroxide. Just substitute ½ of the amount of bleach with peroxide or mix washing soda and water into a paste to pre-treat stains before washing. (Be sure to wear gloves.) Non-chlorine bleach made by Seventh Generation is also available at health food and some regular grocery stores. When possible, place clothes in the sun after bleaching.

Baking soda is a natural cleaning replacement and can be mixed with water or vinegar for cleaning sink stains and clearing slow drains. Washing soda is another helpful natural cleaner, and the original Bon Ami is a wonderful bath and kitchen cleaner found at the grocery or health food store. (The Bon Ami cleaner and bar are better tolerated than the cleanser.) To naturally disinfect counters use vinegar and water or mix Borax with one gallon of water. Many new products for cleaning the home are available at health food stores and through catalogs. *Or, refer to* Less Toxic Living *(one of the first books to offer alternative safe ways of cleaning) and/or* Naturally Clean. *See Resources.* Remember, it's best to limit the amount of different products you use in your home. Less is considered best.

> *Avoid conventional latex gloves. Some Whole Foods Markets carry a brand of gloves called True Blues that are a safer alternative to the irritating gloves found at regular grocery and drug stores.*

While cleaning and especially vacuuming, wear a mask to filter out the inhalants of common allergies, such as dust and mold. If vacuuming is always a problem, try using special vacuum cleaner bags that capture allergenic particles or buy a vacuum cleaner with a built-in HEPA filter system. HEPA stands for high-efficiency particulate air filtration. These vacuums are offered in some commercial stores or through specialty catalogs such as N.E.E.D.S. *See Resources.* Always let a company know that you are chemically sensitive.

Masks and Respirators

Masks and respirators are designed for different purposes. Some masks are helpful to those with dry sinuses, because they retain moisture from the mouth. Some are made to block pollen, mold, and dust, but aren't intended to block toxic fumes. These masks may instead trap odors and fumes. Special masks with charcoal inserts should be used to block chemical fumes.

Like everything else, masks may be made of irritating synthetic material. Researching different masks and respirators for your individual needs is necessary. Companies such as N.E.E.D.S and AEHF offer consultation to their customers. Some patients with MCS like the organic masks with coconut filters made by Sandra DenBraber, R.N. She offers a variety of styles and materials. *Refer to chemicalinjury.net.*

Pesticides

It is very important to avoid exposure to toxic pest control in your environment. Replace insecticide sprays, no-pest strips, moth balls, crystals, and mothproofed paper. They are very toxic. Natural insect repellents such as cedar wood and chips can also irritate those with chemical sensitivity. Replace pest control with alternative products. Minor problems can occasionally be solved with the laundry booster Borax (found in the detergent section in the grocery). Borax sprinkled in cracks and crevices can help to ward off silverfish and eliminate ants and roaches when mixed with sugar (keep away from children and pets). A mask should be worn while applying Borax to avoid inhaling the dust. (Some patients may be sensitive to Borax.) Oils, such as eucalyptus, as well as hedge apples, can be used to chase away some spiders. Ants usually run away from dried peppermint, cayenne, cucumber skins, tomato vines, and salt. Roaches also don't like cucumber skins and bay leaves.

When pest infestations are serious and pesticides must be used, leave until you feel entirely comfortable and experience no side effects upon returning. However, all patients should avoid organophosphates (OPs), carbamates, and pryrethroids, as well as mulch that contains fungicides or cedar. Because chemicals linger in environments, always inquire when buying an older home if it has been treated with the pesticide called Chlordane. This toxic pesticide can last for decades.

In the garden, try to fight pests and diseases with garlic sprays (if tolerated), safe insecticide soaps, or use Safer Brand, Planet Natural, and /or refer to Gardens Alive! *See Resources.* Be preventive and plant some marigolds in your garden to repel certain insects. Also try "companion planting" (planting different species of plants side by side) to attract beneficial insects. Even Ladybugs can be ordered to reduce certain infestations.

Although you may be able to avoid using chemicals in your garden, you may be affected if you live near a golf course or park. To avoid the toxic effects of these areas find out if and when they are sprayed for insects and how the grass is maintained. Stay away at these times.

Foods Treated with Pesticides

The effects from foods treated with pesticides may not be, at first, as obvious to those with chemical sensitivity. This is because symptoms can often be delayed. Eating foods that have been grown organically is ideal. Generally, organic foods contain two-thirds fewer pesticide residues than foods exposed to pesticides. However, another concern for some patients is sulfur. It's also important for patients to avoid farm grown vegetables sold at stands close to busy roadways because they are exposed to carbon monoxide. It's best to find a farm or natural indoor market that labels ingredients and can answer questions about products.

When buying the following foods, go for organic because these foods are the most affected by synthetic pesticides and fertilizers: spinach, winter squash, bell and hot peppers, potatoes, green beans, celery, pears, peaches, grapes (imported), nectarines (imported), strawberries, blueberries, red raspberries, apples, cherries, nectarines, and wheat. When growing your own vegetables, always check your soil for lead content before planting.

Atrazine, which is a pesticide used heavily on corn and soy, should be avoided. Organic corn and soy do not contain atrazine.

IC/BPS patients, who can tolerate a little coffee, should stick to organic beans. Conventional coffee beans are heavily treated with pesticides. As for alcohol, people with MCS often find that it makes them feel worse, but those who can tolerate a little alcohol should preferably choose vodka. Vodka is not only the purest form of alcohol, it is also available in organic brands, such as Liquid ICE, Crop Organic Vodka, Ocean Vodka, Rain Vodka, Vodka 14, and Square One (100 percent rye and may be irritating).

For information on the health effects of pesticides refer to the National Pesticide Telecommunications Network and regional foundations listed in Resources. For chemical-free pest control refer to Resources.

Patients and everyone, actually, should avoid irradiated food and food that has been genetically engineered. Foods that have been irradiated either have the international Radura symbol (which looks like two leaves under a sun within a broken circle) or the words "treated by irradiation." Unfortunately, sometimes the ingredients in foods may be treated by irradiation without any information, but these ingredients are often found in processed foods that IC/BPS and MCS patients usually avoid. Genetically-engineered or genetically-modified foods (which are altered to be more resistant to pests) are banned in Europe and other countries. In the United States it is up to industry to self-police the standards of foods. However, the International Federation for Produce has designated the number "8" as the first digit of the PLU code for genetically-modified (GM) food. Still, the code is only voluntary and patients should not assume that if the number "8" isn't in the PLU code that the food is not genetically-modified. Rather, patients should look for the NON GMO Project symbol: a butterfly between two leaves. Although it is not always used, the number "9" is designated as the first digit for organic foods. Organic foods are not genetically-modified. Symptoms of GM foods may range from brain fog to fatigue, and GM foods perhaps promote allergies. There really is not much known about the effects of GM foods, but patients with MCS probably experience some symptoms.

Meat, eggs, and dairy products from animals that have been treated with hormones and antibiotics, and have been caged should also be considered. Organic meat, eggs, and dairy products come from animals fed only on grain, grass, or hay (not GM corn) and they contain no growth hormones or antibiotics. Look for the USDA certified-organic label, or the American grass-fed logo for beef. Eating clean foods for your health is expensive but so are health problems. Most IC/BPS patients save money that they would otherwise spend on vitamins and supplements if they could tolerate them.

Patients should refer to the *Green Guide*'s chart on the *Natural Home and Garden* website, naturalhomeandgarden.com, to avoid high levels of mercury, PBDEs, and other contaminants, such as polychlorinated bisphenyls (PCBs) in fish. Patients can also refer to www.epa.gov/ost/fish.

Fish and shellfish, as well as meat and dairy products, often contain the chemical hormone disrupter called dioxin. This is another reason to eat healthy.

Canned Goods

Silicone is sometimes used in the cleaning process of commercial canned cooked vegetables. Although the vegetables are rinsed off after cleaning, some studies have led researchers to suspect that there is harmful residue left on the vegetables. Vegetables, soda, and beer in cans are also exposed to silicone linings. These facts may make eating fresh vegetables and drinking from glass bottles a priority for some patients.

Plastic and Foods

Because some plastic containers contaminate food and drinks with toxins, such as bisphenol A (BPA) and benzene, it's best to follow the *Green Guide's Plastic Picks*. To do so, turn plastic containers or bottles upside down to locate the number in the recycling logo. If the number is a 3, 6, or 7 do not eat or drink from the container or store food in it. If the numbers are 1, 2, 4, or 5 the plastic is considered safe. (Some experts question the numbers 4 and 5.)

Other safety tips form the *Green Guide* are:
- Never reuse plastic water bottles (Instead use a stainless steel bottle, such as a Klean Kanteen, kleankanteen.com, for your drinking water.)
- Never use abrasive cleaners on plastic containers
- Never use plastic wrap, plastic containers, or conventional paper towels in the microwave (Instead use ceramic, microwave-safe glass or non-chlorinated paper towels from Seventh Generation. When using plastic wrap for other purposes always choose BPA-free wrap. Glad offers this plastic wrap.)
- Never use plastic garbage bags that are scented or block odor

When using wax paper choose natural brands, such as If You Care, which contains vegetable wax.

Ventilation and Good Air Quality

Airtight homes are not good for anyone. Proper ventilation is necessary to clear the air of chemicals and control the climate. Although it's important to use proper ventilation at all times, opening windows to outdoor air can often be worse or just not sufficient to clean inside air. People who need to remove organic substances such as mold, dust, and pet dander can use a free-standing HEPA filter to clean the air of particulates (some MCS patients do not do well with HEPA filters). Specialized air filters with activated carbon are available to those who need to remove fumes and odors (toxic pollutants). All people and especially those with impaired immune systems, asthma, and lung problems should avoid ozone machines for cleaning the air. *For specifics about HEPA, specialized air filter systems, and different charcoal filters, contact N.E.E.D.S. See Resources.*

Another way to clean environmental air is with an electrostatic filter placed on the central air return. Electrostatic filters can remove small particles of airborne irritants such as mold, bacteria, and animal dander, as well as keep indoor air clean during heavy traffic or pollen season when windows are usually shut. However, it's necessary to clean an electrostatic filter at least every two weeks. This is especially needed in damp climates in order to keep the air flow free and strong enough to reduce moisture.

Your environment is not always easy to control. Carbon monoxide and other fumes can travel through walls, pipes, floors, cracks, under doors, and, of course, through badly sealed windows and doors. Attached garages may allow carbon monoxide to travel into the home even when garage doors are open.

Venting systems should be checked regularly and furnace filters should be kept clean. Flue gases should also be checked, as well as venting systems and connections. Always check oil burners that smell oily, and check all gas burners, ovens, and appliances. Keep outside grills away from your house, and gas water heaters housed separately when possible. (When grilling with briquettes, use Green Hearts Natural Charcoal Briquettes which are carbon-neutral: greenheartsbriquettes.com. Or, use Cowboy's All Natraul Hardwood Lump Charcoal: cowboycharcoal.com.) Try to avoid gas ovens and appliances. Gas appliances make breathing difficult for people with asthma and/or MCS. Be sure to check them often if you use them. Keep fireplaces clean and open, or close off the chimney and fireplace if they are irritating. Be sure that your clothes dryer vent is clean, clear, and vented outside. Consult a mechanical engineer if ventilation problems arise.

> There is a specific type of MCS that is caused by carbon monoxide poisoning. It is called muses syndrome. Symptoms are not only triggered by chemicals and molds, they are triggered by almost everything. Like typical MCS, patients with muses syndrome react to sensory stimuli such as light (especially fluorescent) and sound, but their reactions are to all types of sensory stimuli. Muses syndrome causes a deficiency that may be reversed with the standard treatment for CO poisoning. Contact MCS Referral and Resources for treatment and prevention of low-level carbon monoxide exposure. See Resources.

It's necessary for the MCS patient to use good ventilation in the kitchen. Smoke from frying and baking can affect breathing. Keeping the oven clean and free of grease is necessary. Cooking with organic foods can also help, because chemicals in foods are actually released during the heating process. (Some patients with MCS like the Jenn-Air ovens because they vent outside.) Everyone should avoid pots and pans with nonstick coating as well, because they contain the carcinogenic chemicals polytetrafluoroethylene (PTFF) and perfluorooctanoic acid (PFOA). In their place, use nonstick ceramic or enamel-coated cast iron.

Eliminating the Items that Expose You to Chemicals in Your Environment

Even with good ventilation, if you have MCS it is necessary to eliminate furniture that contains formaldehyde or deteriorating foam. It is best to replace old foam furniture and buy solid wood or metal furniture instead. The following furniture contains formaldehyde which MCS patients usually react to very quickly, especially when the furniture is new:

- Furniture made from particleboard
- Furniture made from plywood (unless the plywood has been made without formaldehyde)
- Medium-density fiberboard

Carpeting and its padding can be a big source of volatile organic chemicals (VOCs) that release formaldehyde, toluene, and xylene. If you can tolerate some carpeting in your home use all cotton, nylon, or untreated wool Persian or Chinese carpets. (Natural jute may need to be avoided.) Always double check treatments and avoid carpets that have been treated with a bactericide or a fumigant. Check for synthetic backings, which may contain synthetic latex and/or irritating adhesives. Use only plain felt carpet pads or cotton fiber. Steam should be used to clean carpets and not carpet soaps, unless they are organic and scent-free. When installing wall-to-wall carpet be sure to have the carpet tacked down and not glued down. If possible have the carpet aired-out before installation. If carpeting has been water damaged, it must be replaced. Remember carpets collect VOCs, dust, fragrances, and other irritants, so it's important to vacuum often and use good ventilation.

Paints, plastics, adhesives, carpets, and furniture, as well as other products, can out-gas the toxic chemical toluene. Refer to HealthyStuff.org to find ratings on everyday products from children's toys to cars.

Other environmental hazards include:

- Furniture treated with stain guard. (When possible order new upholstered furniture without stain guard. Ask the company if they will remove the plastic covering and store your new piece of furniture away from chemicals for a

couple of weeks until it out-gasses. Slip covers are easier to maintain.)
- Treated leather furniture (All leather absorbs fragrance, even leather seats in cars.)
- Rubber foam cushions
- Furniture with deteriorating foam

It's very important to avoid fumes and odors while you are sleeping. Become aware of the smaller items and products in your bedroom that may affect you:

- Newsprint
- Strong inks or mold in books
- New computer tablets
- Glues and tapes

When you don't need your sales receipts, have the cashier, sales person, or waiter throw them away. Many cash register receipts contain BPA.

Climate Control

Controlling the humidity in your environment is essential to fight health problems. In the winter months sinuses can become dry and irritated, which can result in increased susceptibility to odors and illness, particularly for MCS patients with sensitive mucous membranes.

Steam radiators are preferable to dry forced air, which can be very irritating to the sinuses. Most people benefit from the use of a humidifier in the winter months; however, it's necessary to keep humidifiers away from carpeting so it does not become wet. Humidifiers can be placed on tables if necessary. They should be cleaned often with a little vinegar and water. Some experts say that the humidity in your home should not get higher than 50 percent, if possible. Others say 35 percent. A humidity gauge can be used to check and control levels.

When the humidity gets too high, other problems arise. In the summer months an air conditioner (which is a dehumidifier) and/

or a free-standing dehumidifier can help to cut down humidity. Filters and ducts must stay clean and free of mold and mildew. Air return filters should be cleaned every couple of weeks. Air ducts need cleaning at least every ten years, and perhaps more often in damper climates, but avoid using fungicides and harsh chemicals. Look for non-toxic solutions to remove and prevent mildew.

HVAC stands for a good heating, ventilating, and air conditioning system, which brings outside air into the house while removing chemicals and filtering impurities. HVAC systems are expensive, but for some, may be worth the cost. Ceiling fans help to move stagnant air, but when air passes over mold, mildew, or a dusty area, it can create problems. Keeping the environment (including vents and fans) clean and properly ventilated is necessary. So is leaving—when and if bleaches or other strong cleaning agents are used—and not returning until the fumes have vanished.

Shared Living

MCS patients who live in apartments or condos often must make modifications. Those who live with shared venting may have to cover their vents with aluminum or Denny Foil to keep occasional strong fumes out. But, when closing off re-circulated air in the winter, it's often necessary to use a portable heater (avoid portable radiators that are filled with oil) or a window air conditioner in the summer. People with MCS need apartment or condo management that is considerate and practices the laws that protect residents under the Fair Housing Act. Residents who are qualified as handicapped can request reasonable accommodations such as being notified before any new work, painting, or pest control is started.

Everyone should automatically be notified before new work begins no matter who they are, but most residents in a shared building are not sensitive to the individual resident's needs. No matter, every person should be aware that well-meaning healthy people in charge of projects can innocently replace unacceptable products without understanding the consequences to a sensitive person.

The Work Space

Work performance can be hindered when chemically sensitive people are exposed to chemicals in the workplace. These following tips may help when they are possible:

- Move your desk away from copy machines and printers (Solvent-based laser printers are more toxic than water-based ink printers.)
- Avoid felt-tip pens and use mechanical pencils if you are sensitive to wood bound pencils
- Avoid instant glues
- Limit exposure to plastics such as some electrical and electronic equipment with heated surfaces (Chemical residues volatilize with heating.)
- Take breaks while using such equipment
- Buy a small special air filter for the workspace
- Avoid carbonless copy paper
- Try to avoid correction fluids, new cardboard, and glossy paper
- Let a new computer, especially a laptop, out-gas for a month or more before using. Another option is to trade your new computer with someone who can lend you an older one for a period of time. This can give the computer time to out-gas metals and toxic chemicals, such as fire-retardants. A better option is to find electronic companies that are phasing out the chemicals in their products. Less-toxic computers are worth researching.

People with chronic fatigue syndrome (CFS) may experience electromagnetic hypersensitivity (EHS). People with chemical sensitivity may also be susceptible to EHS.

There is legal protection for the chemically handicapped at work. Under the Americans with Disabilities Act (ADA), if an employee has a disability that might interfere with job performance, the employer must assess whether it is possible to "reasonably accommodate" the individual on the job. There may be legal recourse if chemicals are a problem in your workplace and no one will listen.

Travel

Travel is already difficult for most IC/BPS patients. When one is also chemically sensitive, the following suggestions can be helpful.

Car Travel

Shut the windows and fresh air vent while driving in heavy traffic or during pollen season. Use the re-circulate vent instead. Be aware of sensitivities to the heater, fan, or defroster (the defroster uses outside air). Sensitive patients might be more comfortable using the air conditioner. The air conditioner can be set to the warmest temperature when necessary. Start the car with the air shut off to avoid fumes and/or a pollen shower. Also avoid squirting the windshield solution with the vents open. Wait until the windshield dries to open the vents.

Another way to improve the air quality in your car is with a small specialized charcoal filter air cleaner. Clean air is important while driving in heavy traffic, driving in a new car, or driving on freshly laid tar. (Get rid of the new car smell with a non-toxic product called Smelleze. Go to www.NoOrdor.com.) Always avoid ozone machines or air filters containing ozone. You do not want to breathe ozone while you are driving, because it may make you lightheaded and confused.

Gasoline, auto exhaust, dashboards, car seats, and strong air fresheners used in cars outgas the toxic chemical benzene. Patients with MCS usually must avoid pumping their own gas.

Plane Travel

Sometimes even entering an airport can be offensive. The strong fumes that accompany air travel can make one nauseated, lightheaded, and create sinus and breathing problems. Inside a plane there is increased exposure to fumes because one is in a small space that has an artificial source of oxygen and furnishings that contain PBDEs. (These chemicals are also used in train furnishings and release in old sofas.) Some people choose to wear special, small fresh air machines around their necks when they travel. Although these necklaces can provide temporary relief, they can contain a small amount of ozone. Ozone is not good for patients with MCS, asthma, and breathing problems. *For information call the AEHF in Resources. For general information on plane travel send for the book* Jet Smarter, *by Diana Fairechild (available on Amazon).*

> *The bowel is known to swell during flight. Perhaps the bladder also swells, because altitudes are known to increase frequency.*

Hotel Stays

Obviously, people with MCS need to stay at non-smoking hotels. (Smoking rooms are still available in some hotels.) Patients should always ask for rooms that have not been cleaned with air fresheners, carpet fresheners, scented sprays, ozone machines, or newly painted, renovated, or carpeted rooms, when making hotel reservations. This request works pretty well with some hotels. And, although there are some hotels that will swab down the room with vinegar, this is rare. So, bring along a plastic spray bottle and some vinegar to neutralize the room. Try to pick hotels with windows that open, or better yet, reserve rooms with sliding glass doors to the outside. You can then request your reserved room be aired in advance. Bring extra pillow cases and your own pillow to avoid strong bleach or scented fumes in bedding. Always place hotel soaps and toiletries in a drawer; they are usually highly scented.

> *Most MCS patients can quickly detect if ozone has been recently used. If it has, the patient can either leave for a period of time while the room airs out, or request a room that has not been recently cleaned.*

Although hotel stays can be challenging, you may be more comfortable staying in a hotel than in a friend's home. It's usually easier to express your needs and/or complaints in a hotel. Some

Marriot Hotels, Hyatt Hotels and Resorts, and Fairmont Hotels and Resorts offer rooms for people with allergies, breathing problems, and MCS. Patients can also refer to safertraveldirectory. com, yellowcanary.com, or travelorganic.com. Of course, patients with severe MCS may not be candidates for hotel stays or even travel.

Some patients who have become ill from chemical exposure or patients who need to leave their environment because of chemicals being used have stayed at the Natural Place. This is a Florida residence with apartments and hotel rooms that caters to people with allergies and chemical sensitivity. Another residence which offers world-class therapies is the Hippocrates Health Institute in West Palm Beach, Florida. Many people are drawn to this institute to recover from various conditions. *Refer to Resources.*

Building or Remodeling a Toxic-Free Home

When building or remodeling, it is essential for people with chemical sensitivity to check all building materials carefully before using. Particleboard, plywood (some of the newer plywood may be made without formaldehyde), and medium-density fiberboard are big sources of formaldehyde. To avoid formaldehyde, ask stores or companies for a copy of the MSDS for product contents. (But even a MSDS does not have to list products not considered toxic by regulators.) Replace plywood with outdoor plywood, wheatboard, formaldehyde-free particleboard, or medium density fiberboard, unless indoor plywood has no formaldehyde. Use solid wood, steel, enamel, or open metal cabinets. Avoid wood veneers and vinyl coated cabinets. Counters should be made of tile, granite, soapstone, concrete, or solid wood.

Avoid treated wood in and outside of the home, including fences. The wet runoff from newly treated wood is toxic to the land, to animals, and to close fishponds.

Use *solid* wood, ceramic tile, natural linoleum, cork, or polished concrete on floors instead of wall-to-wall carpeting and/

or vinyl floors, which contain PVC. Pre-sealed solid wood floors should off-gas less than floors that are sealed after installation. But sealed floors, such as bamboo, may contain formaldehyde, toxic adhesives, and/or a questionable moisture barrier, which all can out-gas as the sealing wears. And although water based urethane, paint or clear resin are considered safe for most people, sensitive patients should consider sealing floors with a safe wax. Patients should also understand that clear varnishes are better than stains, but they still need time to off-gas toxic fumes. *See Resources for the least toxic sealants and varnishes.*

> *Avoid cork tiles with vinyl backing and all flooring containing formaldehyde. Since Marmoleum (natural linoleum) contains pine rosin and jute, it should probably also be avoided. Also cork has a very strong odor.*

Building products need to be well researched for your individual needs. Vinyl window frames can contain chemicals to deter pests and mildew. Window screens may also contain chemicals. Paints can contain ammonia, formaldehyde, benzene, toluene, fungicides and pesticides. Latex, low-odor, low, or zero volatile organic compounds (VOCs) can still produce strong fumes. Oil-based paints should always be avoided, even on the outside of the home unless patients leave for a period of time. The safest paints are specialized plant and milk based (non-petroleum), or clay. Patients can try SafePaint from the Old-Fashioned Milk Paint Company, Mythic Black Label Paint, or clay plaster with mineral pigments. Silicone caulking can also present a problem and the fumes can take time to dissipate or off-gas; however, they are usually better tolerated than latex sealers. Although some caulking may be fast drying, caulking made for windows and doors may be more tolerable than tub caulking. Drywall compound may be okay, but patients may not be able to tolerate wallpaper made of vinyl, and/or find that plain wallpaper causes problems if the glue under the paper mildews. It's usually wise to avoid hanging wallpaper in damp areas and rooms without windows. Using a nontoxic glue and/or tacking for a natural fabric wall covering, such rice paper, silk, linen, or bamboo, is a safer choice. (Wall coverings made of jute and grasses may not be suitable for patients with MCS.) When fiberglass insulation is used, it's important to use formaldehyde-free insulation or, if using insulation containing formaldehyde, it should be contained and wrapped tightly to keep formaldehyde from emitting toxic gases. Seams and joints in insulated duct work can be taped and sealed with a low-odor aluminum foil tape, such as Polyken Tape, to prevent leakage. If possible, always avoid plastic ductwork and have ducts cleaned only with water or an environmentally safe cleanser. Never let a company use toxic fungicides.

New metal duct sheeting must be power washed before installing due to the oil on the sheeting. Vinegar can also help to cut the oil.

Other products used in the home should be considered. Replace duct tape with aluminum tape or stainless steel adhesive tape. Use only white glue like Elmer's Glue or yellow woodworking glue. And, be sure to store all chemicals, including paint, in a separate, well ventilated space.

Plastics, synthetic rubber, and solvents outgas the toxic chemical benzene.

Ideally, your new home or addition should be free of gas appliances and heaters. Solar and electric heat, air conditioning, and appliances are healthier. Most homes can be converted from gas to electricity. If you build a new home or addition, be sure that it is well ventilated with outdoor air supplies to the kitchen, bath, and laundry area. Living well is necessary and often difficult. Recognizing your needs is the first step and taking action is the second and most important step. *To learn more about the potential harm of various chemicals refer to www.scorecard.org.*

New appliances usually need to off-gas. Place vinegar in a new dishwasher's soap panel and run it several times. Swab a new oven with vinegar and baking soda, although it may take time for the oven to out-gas.

Resources

National Multiple Chemical Sensitivity (MCS) Organizations

Human Ecology Action League (HEAL)
(Support groups and newsletters)
www.healnatl.org • (770) 389-4519

National Center for Environmental Health Strategies (NCEHS)
(Newsletters)
www.ncehs.org • (856) 429-5358 • (856) 816-8820

Chemical Injury Information Network (CIIN)
www.ciin.org • (406) 547-2255

Books

(Some of the following books are older but still considered staples for MCS patients.)

Toxic Beauty: Cosmetics and Personal-Care Products Endanger Your Health, Samuel S. Epstein, M.D. and Randall Fitzgerald

Not Just a Pretty Face: The Ugly Side of the Beauty Industry, Stacy Malkan

Less Toxic Living or Less Toxic Alternatives, Carolyn P. Gorman

Naturally Clean: The Seventh Generation Guide to Safe and Healthy, Non-Toxic Cleaning, Jeffrey Hollender, Geoff Davis, and Meika Hollender

Better Basics for the Home: Simple Solutions for Less Toxic Living, Annie Berthold-Bond

Chemical Exposures, Low Levels and High Stakes, Second Edition, Nicholas Ashford and Claudia Miller

Staying Well in a Toxic World: Understanding Environmental Illness, Multiple Chemical Sensitivities, Chemical Injuries, and Sick Building Syndrome, Lynn Lawson

Jet Smarter: The Air Traveler's Rx, Diana Fairechild

Healthy House Building for the New Millennium, John Bower

Information, Consultation, Products, and Supplies

Always indicate that you are ordering for a MCS person and would like your products and wrappings fragrance-free. Inquire about return policies.

American Environmental Health Foundation, Inc. (AEHF)
(air filters, medical supplies, and products)
www.aehf.com • (800) 428-2343• (214) 361-9515

Multiple Chemical Sensitivity (MCS) Referral and Resources
www.mcsrr.org • (410) 889-6666

N.E.E.D.S *(National Ecological and Environmental Delivery Systems)*
(Filters, masks, products, and newsletters)
www.needs.com • (800) 634-1380

Janice Corporation (Organic clothing, cleaning supplies, catalogs)
www.janices.com • (800) 526-4237

AFM Safecoat Paints and Sealants (Dealer locator for products)
www.afmsafecoat.com • (800) 239-0321

Bioshield Healthy Living Paints (Clay plasters and flooring)
www.bioshieldpaint.com • (800) 621-2591

The Healthy Home, Myron and Dave Wentz
www.myhealthyhome.com

Real Goods (Building materials, batteries, solar products, toys,
cleaning products, and more)
www.realgoods.com• (888) 567-6527 (56SOLAR)

Gaiam Living (Sheets, towels, underwear, cleaning products,
filters, and yoga clothes and equipment)
www.gaiam.com • (877) 989-6321

Cozy Pure
www.organiccomfortzone.com • (800) 229-7571

Keetsa Tea Leaf Contour Pillow
www.keetsa.com • (877) 753-3872

Pesticide Information

Beyond Pesticides (formerly The National Coalition Against the
Misuse of Pesticides (NCAMP)
www.beyondpesticides.org • (202) 543-5450

National Pesticide Information Center (Effects of pesticides)
www.nptn.orst.edu • (800) 858-7378 (PEST)

Pesticide Action Network North America
www.panna.org • (510) 788-9020

U.S. Environmental Protection Agency

www.epa.gov/pesticides

A Toxic-Free Home

Healthy House Institute
www.healthyhouseinstitute.com • (208) 724-1508

Build It Green (Green resource center)
www.builditgreen.org
(510) 590-3360 (Northern California)
(213) 688-0070 (Southern California)

Chemical-Free Retreats

The Natural Place Apartments
www.thenaturalplace.com• (954) 428-5438

Hippocrates Institute
www.hippocratesinst.org • (888) 228-1755

Chapter Seven

IDENTIFYING, CONTROLLING, AND AVOIDING IC/BPS SYMPTOMS WITH SELF-HELP

Pain Is Motivation to Change

Almost every IC/BPS patient will agree that they would rather go through anything else but the pain of a bad IC/BPS flare-up. While it's normal for new patients to first wonder why and how they got interstitial cystitis/bladder pain syndrome, as they become engrossed in the process of finding a successful treatment, their focus usually changes to recognizing and identifying the particular factors and culprits that set off their symptoms.

With the right knowledge, IC/BPS patients quickly learn to understand their painful flare-ups and even sometimes predict their durations as they become more familiar with this disease. Unfortunately, there are still many helpful suggestions that patients may overlook when they do not need help for a particular symptom. The following tips are intended to give more control to individuals who learn to turn to themselves for relief and prevention.

Coping with Urgency and Frequency

Two self-help techniques for IC/BPS patients who experience urgency and frequency are bladder training and double voiding.

Bladder Training

When you need to use the bathroom to void, and there isn't one around, you use your bladder sphincter muscles to hold your urine. Your sphincter muscles are controlled by voluntary type nerves. When your bladder expands because of the amount of urine stored in it, the traction on your bladder wall elicits a reflex of fullness. This reflex is an involuntary-nervous-system controlled function. But, if you have IC/BPS, you may experience a false fullness in your bladder meaning that there is not enough urine in your bladder to warn the involuntary or reflex response that helps you urinate when your bladder is full. A vicious cycle results in urgency, frequency, and poor emptying caused by muscle damage. The damage occurs from frequently voiding a bladder that isn't able to hold a small amount of urine without pain, pressure, and/or frequency (a normal bladder holds about a pint of urine for a couple of hours). However, bladder training can help to strengthen your bladder muscle, improve circulation, and increase your bladder capacity, all of which may restore a more comfortable voiding pattern. With practice, you will usually experience improvement in several weeks.

Experts advise IC/BPS patients to add a few minutes to their intervals between voiding in order to retrain the bladder nerves and muscles, and increase bladder capacity. Obviously this protocol should not be practiced while one is in pain or experiencing the first challenges of IC/BPS. And, like other treatments, it may not be right for every patient. Some IC/BPS patients find distraction the best tool to use while lengthening interval times.

Everyone with IC/BPS has experienced a situation when they have had to hold urine just a little longer than they would like. When this occurs, their urine stream often becomes stronger when they finally void. They also may find they can empty their bladder more fully, and sometimes do not feel the urge to void again as soon. The longer interval has actually helped their bladder to function better.

However, the opposite can happen when patients who suffer with frequency and urgency have had to wait so long that they experience pain. When this happens, there may be difficulty beginning a urine stream or fully voiding. In this case the bladder has become distended (this can happen overnight as well), which can be very painful and cause spasms. Bladder training needs to be practiced slowly and comfortably in order to strengthen the urine stream, reduce urgency, and help to calm a frequency cycle. Bladder training is best used in conjunction with medications and other treatments for IC/BPS.

Double Voiding

Patients who have the urgency to void again right after they urinate usually cannot void fully. Even the smallest amount of urine can be an irritant, add pressure, and create the urgent need to empty the bladder again. By taking time after finishing a urine stream to void a second time, most IC/BPS patients find they can empty their bladders more fully, and therefore, reduce the pressure that creates the urgency to void again.

If you try double voiding, wait several seconds after you have completed your first void, relax, and then without straining, try to void again. Use different methods to encourage a second void, such as deep breathing, visualization, shifting your sitting position, stretching your upper body, or picking up a magazine to shift your mind away from the task. The toilet is also a safe place to try deep breathing into your belly without the worry that you will have to get up to go void.

There are two methods that may be used to help empty a stubborn bladder. One is the Credé maneuver, which is done by applying pressure to the lower abdomen with hands facing each other and fingers spread, somewhat overlapping. The other method is the Valsalva maneuver, which requires bending forward over the thighs to create pressure on the lower abdomen before voiding. The Valsalva method may be more comfortable for IC/BPS patients. These methods were probably invented by someone with bladder symptoms because many patients naturally use these methods to rid irritating urine.

Although these methods can work, double voiding without straining is the safest and the healthiest way to empty your bladder. The pressure used in the Credé maneuver and the Valsalva maneuver can force urine back up into the ureters in some people. IC/BPS patients who have acid reflux may also not be candidates for these maneuvers.

Patients who suffer with urinary retention sometimes use an intermittent catheter to void their irritating urine. The same type of catheter is used when patients self-catheterize to instill medications. Home catheters are about six inches long and come in different sizes. Smaller sizes, such as pediatric catheters, seem to be more comfortable for patients but they take longer to deliver medication. Larger sized catheters mean less dwelling time, but may be uncomfortable. Lidocaine gel is often applied to the outside of the urethra, placed inside the urethra or on the tip of the catheter to make insertion easier and less painful. But patient preference is individual with catheterization and there are patients who find that lidocaine irritates their bladders.

Aside from the diameter of a catheter, there are different shapes and lengths, and flexibility, as well as materials to choose from. (In certain instances male patients may choose to use a condom catheter.) Catheters are typically made of latex rubber or silicone, Teflon or polyvinylchloride (PVC). Some catheters contain lubricants or antibacterial coatings. Because so many IC/BPS patients have allergies and/or sensitivities, all of these options should be carefully reviewed with a health professional. For instance, a patient who is sensitive to latex may want to use a latex-free LoFric Catheter made by Astra Tech. Although self-catheterization gives many patients a sense of control, it poses a risk of infection. Patients must always use sterile precautions.

For more information on catheters, supplies, instilled medications and insurance coverage refer to the ICA and the IC Network.

Painful Flare-ups

Although patients become acutely attentive to their IC/BPS management, they may find that controlling the symptoms of IC/BPS is like playing the children's game, "Mother May I." Symptoms can get out of control and flare-ups can just happen.

The disease, the bladder pain, and the management of IC/BPS are different for each patient. Depending on the individual some pain may be managed in a few hours or overnight. But there are times when bladder pain develops into a nasty flare-up. When this happens, the flare-up has all of the individual's attention, controlling both mind and body.

IC/BPS flare-ups may involve pressure, urgency, frequency, burning, stinging, urethral, bladder, and pelvic floor spasms, as well as pain in the vagina (or penis and scrotum), perineum, and/or rectum. Patients may experience referred low back and leg pain, and a feeling of weakness and shakiness in their torso, hips, and/or legs. Some patients also describe a pulling sensation in their pelvic floor and an overall experience of feeling held up in a tension pattern. IC/BPS symptoms have been compared to having a knife turning in the bladder, ground glass in the bladder, a lit match, an ant pile, a bladder migraine, a relentless nagging sensation, dryness, soreness, and a throbbing feeling.

Although symptoms vary from patient to patient, everyone affected can agree that when the pain comes, it's like having a dark veil dropped over the spirit. Everything can look and feel different the minute the pain begins. A patient may feel as if she or he has been taken from the present surroundings, isolated, and shut down. This experience can happen very quickly, and cause fear and anxiety about the next moment, future responsibilities, expectations, and duration of the pain.

Pain leads to changes in the central nervous system. There is a great need to act quickly, and to deal with the present as a *fight or flight* reaction takes place in the body. Figuring how and why the pain has happened is normal. A flare-up is a very big disappointment to the IC/BPS patient and often to those around her or him. Feelings of guilt or self-blame can make the reaction to the pain worse. The focus must be on pain relief. Pain is never healthy, even in minimal amounts. Pain is a signal to do something quickly to stop it, and ultimately, to stop doing something that may be causing it.

Treating a Flare-Up

IC/BPS patients treat and cope with their flare-ups in different ways. Some patients need to retire and put their feet up when IC/BPS symptoms begin to flare. Most patients drink a lot of water to dilute their urine or wash away the irritant. But, there are other patients who must quit forcing water in order to stop the pressure, bloating, and the nonstop urgency and frequency. Baking soda (one teaspoon in a glass of water) or Prelief is helpful to neutralize stomach acid, which affects IC/BPS. Eating every three to four hours is also essential to reduce stomach acid and hydrate the body. Of course, many patients must take medications immediately or may need a combination of treatments to treat a flare-up.

The following information details various problem-solving and coping techniques that IC/BPS patients use to treat the different degrees and symptoms of a flare-up.

Reclining to Relieve IC/BPS and Associated Muscle Weakness

Feeling weakness and shakiness in your muscles is a signal which tells you that you are overextending yourself. Weakness and shakiness should also be a cue for you to get off your feet and lie down so that you can relieve the tension in your postural muscles. Although your body will be fully supported while you are lying down, you will need additional support for your upper back, neck, head, and arms if you read or watch TV. Using a bed wedge may be helpful. You can usually find these large wedges in stores or catalogs specializing in products for your back. For optimum support when using a bed wedge, place a pillow under your head and another one on your stomach to support your arms and a book if you are reading. The angle of the wedge should place your abdominal muscles in slack and allow them to rest. The longer the bed wedge is, the better for your body. If your bed wedge puts pressure on your sacrum and tailbone, add a small flat folded towel to make the wedge longer. Other bedding products that can be used for sitting up in bed are the Comfort Reader Pillow and the Hypoallergenic Flex-Arm Bed Lounge found at The Vermont Country Store. *Refer to Resources in Chapter Five.*

When you need to rest flat on the bed, try a jack knife position. Turn on your side and bring your legs straight out in front of you. This position will put your abdominal muscles in slack and stretch out your low back, buttocks, and hamstring muscles. You can also stretch your hip flexors (which is very important) in this position by bringing one leg straight under your body while leaving the other straight out in front. To increase this stretch, bend your knees. No matter how you relieve a flare-up, make sure that you incorporate proper support for your body while you're in a tension pattern.

Cold and Heat Therapy for Bladder Spasms and Burning

Typically the rule is cold for inflammation and heat for muscle spasms. Cold constricts the blood vessels which reduces the flow of blood to the area and helps to slow the body's response to inflammation. IC/BPS patients, however, seem to vary in their preferences. Some women reduce bladder pain and burning by holding a cold pack just above the clitoris for 15 to 20 minutes. Relief is often not felt until the cold pack is lifted away. Some patients may prefer to avoid contact with the sensitive genital areas while using cold packs. Wrapping the cold pack with a thick towel can make the pack more comfortable, as well as prevent frostbite.

Other IC/BPS patients find relief by placing a cold or hot pack on the perineum area between the anus and vagina (between the anus and base of the penis in men) to relieve bladder pain. Female patients who are prone to yeast infections may not be candidates for heat in this area. Some patients prefer to use heat on their low back or abdomen, or use a heated mattress pad to relieve the whole body effect of IC/BPS pain. It's important to be cautious because too much heat is not good for inflammation. Moist heat is best for the bladder and pelvic floor. Both hot and cold packs should last the appropriate therapeutic time, about 20 minutes. Hot packs should not be replaced again for another two hours.

IC/BPS patients who find relief with pelvic floor cold packs can make their own packs by following these wonderful suggestions from other patients:

- Fill a tube sock with rice. Seal the top of the sock and freeze it. Place the frozen pack on your pelvic floor or just above your clitoris. Check the materials used in the tube sock to avoid irritation when the pack starts to melt. Patients with sensitivity to fragrance should avoid pre-made rice packs that contain fragrance.

- Pour water on a heavy flow fragrance-free maxi-pad. Then place the pad in a bowl so it bends and contours to your pelvis after it is frozen. Be sure to wrap the pad well before application.

A Perineal Cold Pack (found at the IC Network), TheraCare HeatWraps (found at drug stores), and Bodi Heat Stick-on Pads (available at the IC Network) have also helped patients to calm symptoms. A product called EndoFemm, which conforms to the pelvic girdle to relieve many pelvic conditions, offers both hot and cold relief to IC/BPS patients. EndoFemm can be ordered from Desert Harvest.

The benefits of hot and cold are not entirely limited to external use. Drinking a hot beverage in the morning can relax the bladder muscle and help to dilute concentrated urine. Eating cold ice cream helps some patients during a flare-up. Of course, hot and cold drinks and food must be bladder-safe for the individual. Experience and preference is unique to each IC/BPS patient.

If neutralizing stomach acids is helpful, try Prelief or a teaspoon of baking soda in water. Or, ask your doctor for a prescription for Tagamet. (Tagamet has been known to create bladder pain in some IC/BPS patients.) Remember to eat every three to four hours to reduce stomach acids and stay hydrated. *See Chapter Two for more information.*

Relieving Bladder Spasms with a Bladder Massage

A bladder massage may not sound very comfortable, but it can help to calm uncomfortable spasms. This massage technique is best performed by a partner or a massage therapist. It is very simple. Following the top edge of the pubic bone (the bone in front of the bladder) from one side to the other, make small, circular massage strokes upward toward the belly with two or three fingers. Repeat these strokes as many times as needed and increase or decrease pressure as needed, then massage the tight areas on each side of the bone where the legs join. Follow these tight areas down and then upward toward the hips.

The bladder massage can help to relax a contracted bladder as well as the surrounding muscles. This technique works very well in conjunction with medication, or for some patients, alone. Massage work in general can be helpful in breaking a tension pattern.

With the help of a trained physical therapist, patients can also learn to release their own bladder, pelvic floor, and abdominal trigger points. (Patients can try the Syracuse Medical Vaginal Dilation for home use: 800-382-5879.) Trigger points in the bladder, pelvic floor, and abdomen can be responsible for pressure, urgency, frequency, and pain (and sometimes infection). Patients with FMS and/or wide-spread IC/BPS can refer to *The Trigger Point Therapy Workbook*. This thorough reference guide, by Clair Davies, N.C.T.M.B., helps patients to identify trigger points (MTrPs) throughout their bodies, understand how these MTrPs contribute to their pain patterns, and learn how to treat them. Although fingers usually work just fine, some people like to use different tools to release MTrPs. These include:

- Trigger Point Pro which has a reflexology tip
- Thera Cane which is used for deep-pressure massage (and is very popular with FMS patients)
- Backnobber used for pain-releasing pressure
- Trigger Point Tools to release soft tissue trigger points
- T-Bar and L-Bar for stimulating trigger points

To order the Thera Cane and/or the other tools, refer to www. theracane.com or www.MassageWarehouse.com.

When Flare-ups Turn into Pain Cycles

Scheduling a Treatment or Appointment

When there is little relief from a flare-up day after day, many IC/BPS patients call their urologists or urogynecologists to schedule a treatment or ask for a new medication.

It's necessary to have a doctor who offers immediate treatment, especially for the patient who depends on bladder instillations for relief. As any IC/BPS patient knows, symptoms are often unpredictable and flare-ups can be a surprise. The ideal doctor will believe you, encourage your IC/BPS management, and give you positive feedback, as well as relief. The IC/BPS patient needs a doctor who can accept the whole picture of her or his illness. Unfortunately, this doesn't always happen.

Many patients with chronic conditions get negative responses from doctors so they learn to edit or hold back information. Chronic pain patients often must seek approval to get help. However, patients with the pain of IC/BPS cannot spare a moment to get another person's approval. Insisting on immediate care will not work with many doctors, but if IC/BPS patients are too calm, their pain may not be recognized or treated. Office visits can end up seeming like a balancing act. Receptionists and doctors who do not understand IC/BPS may see patients as extremely emotional. This includes some urologists and urogynecologists. Most IC/BPS patients can get oral medications from other doctors, such as primary care physicians, if they cannot find the right urologist. Patients not dependent on urologists for treatments may do better by working with other doctors who are available to their needs.

Contact another IC/BPS Patient

Avoid suffering in silence. It's easy to lose perspective when you are in IC/BPS pain. Another IC/BPS patient will understand, remind you that you will feel better and often give you helpful suggestions. Being able to communicate your symptoms, and express how they make you feel may help to begin a healing process. Staying in touch with another patient while you seek medical help can also be reassuring and empowering. No one else can understand your situation as well as another IC/BPS patient. Living with IC/BPS requires support and psychological resilience.

When Pain Cycles Cause More Stress in Your Life

After a few days of pain a person's whole body takes on a tension pattern. It is very important to try to release this tension, because it can create a vicious cycle that in turn will increase your IC/BPS pain. If you are worn-out from pain, it is vital to eliminate extra stress. Taking time out will make it possible to take strong medications when they would otherwise interfere with typical everyday functions. On a more normal day, work and daily routines may serve as helpful distractions, but taking time out for yourself when you're in a lot of pain is necessary both physically and mentally. It is very important to accept the fact that you will experience down days and will need backup help just for these times.

Get Out of Your Environment

A stubborn pain cycle is a vicious cycle. If you have been house bound and your pain isn't improving, it's sometimes necessary to get out of your environment. Get dressed, put on make-up or whatever you usually do before going out, and then leave the house for a little while. You may benefit from a change of scenery. Because change can help you to feel a shift in your emotions, it can have a positive physical effect in breaking a pain cycle. Getting involved and participating in something a little different can also help.

Fatigue the Pain Pattern

For some patients the only way to beat the pain of IC/BPS is to match it, wear it down. The false energy or hyper feeling some IC/BPS patients experience with their bladder pain can cause them to pace. When one finds it difficult to sit still, is exhausted from the tension in her or his body, and cannot find relief with medication or relaxation techniques, it sometimes works to fatigue the muscles naturally through appropriate movement.

One way to fatigue muscles is by walking at a fast pace (not power walking). Taking a short walk close to home can also help to break a frequency cycle. Patients who are unable to walk because of the impact to their bladders may want to try other forms of movement. Stretching and free-form dancing, a dance video, or another form of comfortable exercise done in your home can serve as an alternative. Turn on music. Music is movement and can help to cycle patients out of a pattern. The goal of movement is to fatigue the pain, to tire out the pattern in the muscles, to increase circulation, encourage full breathing, and produce endorphins, which can help to repair the effect IC/BPS has on the limbic system.

Recognizing Your Pain Triggers

When you can't pinpoint the cause of an ongoing pain pattern, it can be frustrating to try to make sense of it or find a way to stop it. But you can help yourself by reviewing the different culprits reported as pain triggers by IC/BPS patients. If you can pinpoint and make yourself aware of your triggers, you can hopefully stop, better cope with, and prevent some future flare-ups.

Various pain triggers:
- Diet changes, including drinking water and ice (Be aware that city tap water changes periodically in chlorine content and is susceptible to chemical spills.)
- Adverse reactions to medications
- Menstrual cycle
- Perimenopause and menopause
- Stress
- Overextending yourself physically or emotionally
- Sexual activity
- Changes in dietary tolerance
- Lack of restorative sleep
- Urinary tract infection (There may be residue bladder pain from the antibiotic after the infection is healed.)
- Yeast infection
- Dehydration
- Adverse reactions to new therapies
- Adverse reactions to new exercise or exercise that contracts the pelvic floor
- New activities including house and yard work
- Travel
- Adverse reactions to new environments, chemicals, paints, home improvements, pesticides, gasoline, etc.
- Seasonal changes, weather changes
- Poor ergonomics, lack of good support while active or resting
- Tight pants that pull your hips back and under when sitting, or pants and tights that hold your buttocks too close together

Improving the Quality of Your Sleep

IC/BPS patients usually wake-up during the night with pressure, urgency, frequency, and/or pain. Just shifting positions or turning over in bed can trigger a trip to the bathroom, and trying to go back to sleep means having to begin the whole sleep cycle over again before reaching the important stage of restorative sleep.

Here is a look at the different stages of sleep. It takes about an hour and a half to cycle through all of them:

- **Stage one** is considered the lightest level of sleep. During this stage our muscles relax as our temperature drops. We get drowsy and start to drift. Our brain generates fast alpha waves (awake-like brain waves). Jumping, jerking, and a feeling of falling may occur. These activities are sometimes called "sleep start."
- **Stage two** is a transition stage. Waves of electrical activity in our brains slow down, as do our heart rate and our breathing.
- **Stages three and four are deep sleep,** when our brain waves become large and slow down as they turn into delta waves (slow-wave sleep), and our bodies start to shut out stimulation. This is our deepest sleep, which is restorative and vital for many body functions to work well, such as the regulation of our various neurotransmitters and hormones (growth hormone for tissue repair) and substances for recharging our immune system (antibody production). Stages three and four have been combined by the American Academy of Sleep Medicine to just one stage: stage three.
- **The last phase of sleep is REM** (rapid eye movement) and is the dreaming stage of sleep. Our muscles become paralyzed and more relaxed than they were during the deepest level of non-REM sleep. Our eyes flutter and the depth of our breathing increases. Our heartbeat and blood pressure also rise. There is high electrical activity in our brains, similar to our brain waves when we are awake. During our dream

sleep we review our thoughts and events of the day and store them away in our brains.

As mentioned above, our bodies depend on uninterrupted slow-wave sleep (restorative sleep) for the tissue repair of our muscles, our antibody production, the regulation of our different immune system chemicals that fight allergies, bacteria, and viruses, and the regulation of our hormones and neurotransmitters. There have been many studies about the effects of sleep deprivation in FMS patients. For example, the regulation of the stress hormone cortisol is meant to drop during sleep, but the physiologic hyperarousal experienced by FMS and CFS patients during sleep elevates these patient's cortisol levels. (Cortisol is produced by the adrenal glands to promote alertness.) Levels may also be elevated in IC/BPS patients and other people who suffer with severe sleep deprivation. Studies have shown that, when cortisol levels stay high over several months, the hippocampus in the brain can shrink and lead to memory problems, which is sometimes a symptom of FMS. High levels of cortisol production can also lead to an increase in abdominal fat, high blood pressure, insulin resistance, and elevated blood sugar, which increases appetite. People with elevated cortisol levels during sleep may take longer than the average time to reach REM sleep and they may become more susceptible to illness when they experience extra stress and exertion. (Cortisol also reduces levels of glycosaminoglycan.)

Another hormone, called ghrelin, spikes when there is a lack of sleep. Like high levels of cortisol, elevated ghrelin triggers hunger. Lack of refreshing sleep also causes a decrease in a hormone called leptin. Leptin is actually considered the body's natural appetite-suppressor. These hormonal changes explain why people who suffer with sleep deprivation may be susceptible to weight gain. So, it's not only a decrease in physical activity (which usually accompanies the IC/BPS lifestyle) that can lead to weight gain, it's also a lack of hormonal regulation in patients who suffer with sleep deprivation. Exercise and sunlight can help these patients as can eating a small snack consisting of a protein and a carbohydrate before bedtime. Patients with FMS are often advised to try a little nut butter on a cracker before bed to increase sleep without raising blood sugar levels. FMS patients may also try certain supplements, such as melatonin or L-tryptophan to promote and/or maintain sleep, but these supplements are not typically tolerated or helpful to patients with IC/BPS who need help with bladder symptoms.

Sleep deprivation is actually considered a clue to certain diseases. It is a common symptom of interstitial cystitis/bladder pain syndrome, vulvodynia, chronic prostatitis, irritable bowel syndrome, and migraine headaches. It is one of the first signs of fibromyalgia (FMS) and chronic fatigue syndrome (CFS). Although treatment for sleep deprivation in patients with these conditions is usually geared toward pain relief, patients with FMS may also need treatment for certain sleep disorders that can accompany their condition. Treatment for sleep deprivation caused by IC/BPS symptoms is always geared toward reducing pain, because pain and frequency interrupt and prevent sleep. The most effective medications (reviewed in the previous chapters) used to treat sleep deprivation in IC/BPS patients are:

- Elavil (amitriptyline)
- Atarax and Vistaril (hydroxyzine)
- Neurontin (gabapentin)

Some IC/BPS patients choose to take a benzodiazepine, like Valium (diazepam), to fight pain and aid sleep. Sleeping medications such as the hypnotic Ambien (zolpidem) are also often used by patients, but patients should be aware that many medications taken to promote sleep can interfere with the amount of time spent in the different stages of sleep, including restorative sleep. Urologist Robert Moldwin suggests that IC/BPS patients instill anesthetics into their bladders before bed, so symptoms won't keep them awake. They can also perhaps avoid oral medications. But, no matter how a patient encourages sleep, the bottom line is that pain and/or other symptoms in most conditions that cause sleep deprivation increase without restorative sleep.

Illness Breaks the Rules

Dealing with People

Having IC/BPS means dealing with more than physical pain and sleep deprivation. Explaining the effects that IC/BPS has on your life may be one of your hardest challenges, because of the response you get. People who have not been exposed to chronic illness will most probably have a difficult time understanding your pain, needs, and lifestyle.

How well other people understand your IC/BPS can also depend on how well you accept and deal with your own illness. There are many different factors that play into your acceptance of IC/BPS. These factors can include your background, cultural values and beliefs, the role you play in your family, career demands, self-expectations, age, how you've dealt with illness in the past, reactions of family, friends, employers, co-workers, and of course, your doctors. When these factors interfere with your self-care, they are a problem.

IC/BPS requires strict coping skills and it's often necessary to remind the people around you that you have to stay on top of your condition. IC/BPS is invisible to others, but usually, when people spend enough time with you, they find that you are more accessible when you are in control of your own needs. Still at first, you may have to ask for a lot, sift through people and their opinions, and take control before you earn the understanding of those affected by your IC/BPS. Although there may be those who will feel resentful and controlled by your needs, you must remind yourself that you are not responsible for their reactions. If you do not take good care of yourself, you won't be able to take care of anyone or anything else.

You may be often told you lack confidence when you are fearful of taking long car rides, getting in the car with another driver, going to new restaurants, taking trips, or starting new employment. People with this opinion do not understand the complexity of IC/BPS. They do not know how much confidence, willpower, and determination living with IC/BPS takes. Confidence in yourself is a multifaceted issue. You can be completely secure and assertive in certain situations, but not in other situations in which you do not have access to, or know where there's a bathroom that can be reached within a limited time frame.

In general, IC/BPS patients tend to be most confident when they are not rushed and can control their environment in relationship to their bladder needs. When others label an IC/BPS patient as "unconfident" or "not trying," they do not understand this complex disease.

It's essential to educate those around you and make them aware of your unique lifestyle management. You may need to set new boundaries and even make new friends. Learn to represent your new life without being negative. If you can accept your illness, limitations, and modified lifestyle (this does not mean accepting the pain), you will gain admiration and support from most people.

At times, you may have to depend on people you don't care for, such as skeptical and difficult health-care professionals, insurance companies, and even friends and family members. Because of this dependence it's essential (when at all possible) to avoid other people who do not believe that you are limited by IC/BPS.

Experiencing a flare-up around challenging people is not unusual. Your body's protective mechanism is telling you to change a situation or leave. Seeking out supportive people who understand and accept you is necessary, because if you don't feel good about yourself when you're with someone, they are *not good for you!* However, there is a fine line between isolating oneself and protecting oneself from uncomfortable situations and events. Finding new friends may be easier because they will accept you for who you are *now*.

Finding Support

Treating your physical symptoms is the first step of self-help. Treating your emotional pain may be the second. Blame is handed out too easily to victims and at times unconditional love from family and friends isn't there. A good support group can really help this situation. Find a group that actively listens to you and a group that works to improve the quality of life for people with IC/

BPS and other chronic conditions. A good group can offer unconditional support, help you to build a new sense of self-awareness
and control, help you to become assertive and inquisitive, and
perhaps provide you with some nice new friends. All of this will
protect you from the impact of negativity that can exist with IC/
BPS. If you cannot find a local support group, start one by placing
an ad in your paper or get on the internet.

*Barb Zanikow, IC/BPS support group leader and board member
of the ICA, stresses that electronics cannot replace the presence
of another IC/BPS patient.*

In addition to support groups, mental health professionals such as social workers or psychologists can also help you
deal with your disease. Therapists who work with chronic
pain patients have expertise in offering practical lifestyle management strategies, which can help both your physical and
emotional pain. It is important to find a professional who uses
effective counseling, which incorporates dialogue between the
therapist and patient.

It is also necessary to understand the difference between a
psychologist and a psychiatrist when choosing an appropriate
mental health practitioner. A psychiatrist is a medical doctor
with additional training in psychology. Be aware that many psychiatrists have an analytic orientation, which will not meet your
needs if you are looking for a therapist who will actively provide
feedback and suggestions. Psychiatrists, however, have expertise
with psychotropic medications such as antidepressants and anti-
anxiety medications. Consultations with a psychiatrist may help
you find the most effective psychotropic medication with the
fewest side effects.

Successes Improve the Quality of Life

Successes and accomplishments are necessary to achieve a
feeling of involvement and productivity. Without them, life's
problems can become overwhelming and depressing. To achieve
success you first must know yourself and your limitations. You

must accept and understand your unique symptoms to reach your goals realistically. If you learn to manage your time, avoid overextending yourself and seek out safe environments, you can successfully control the daily impact of IC/BPS. When you accomplish more, you will feel a sense of satisfaction.

Successes are more easily achieved when you become more cognizant of your body's tension patterns. When you use proper support and stay physically strong, you can accomplish more. Try to incorporate a comfortable home exercise program. Select music and a comfortable exercise mat. Even if you can only exercise one or two days a week, making the effort will improve the quality of your life, release stress, give you renewed energy, and will reward you with a sense of accomplishment. Success leads to commitment.

Self-Expression Is Necessary

When life's priorities change with IC/BPS, so can your perspective and values. Although the smaller pleasures may take on more meaning for you, you live in an extremely competitive society. You can have a difficult time finding where you fit in, as well as finding your meaning and purpose in our goal oriented world. You may find it necessary to discover new interests and outlets, new forms of escape and ways to express yourself. Because your life has changed so much, you may do this quite successfully. Whether it's painting, drawing, keeping a diary, studying a new topic, pursuing a new hobby or exercise routine, or helping others in need, self-expression is a necessary component to stress management. Self-expression can minimize the mundane chore of dealing with physical problems, as well as affirm your role in society.

Seek Comfort and Make Life Easier

- **Wear comfortable clothes**. Buy slacks a size larger to get more room in the crotch. You can take them in elsewhere. Use scissors and make little downward slits in elastic waist bands to make more room. If you are a woman you can find comfortable, attractive clothes made by Japanese Weekend; and no one needs to know they are designed for pregnancy.

- **Empty your bladder before meals** if you experience frequency and pressure. Eating should not be rushed. You do not need to anticipate a trip to the bathroom.
- **Carry a portable urinal in the car**, even if it's only for peace of mind. The Travel John is very handy and can be used by men, women, and children. Another solution, suggested by Jill Osborne of the ICN, is to keep three towels and a large plastic garbage bag in your car: one towel to cover yourself, one to void into, and the other to clean-up with. Patients who wish to avoid dirty toilet seats or squatting in the outdoors can use GoGirl, a reusable product that assists urination standing up and fits in a purse. Go Girl can be a plus in awkward plane bathrooms. Another option is the Whizzy which also assists standing urination.
- **Carry an ice pack in a freezer bag when travelling** or even better, carry the Cool Water Cone (www.coolwatercone. com) which only needs cold water to chill. Patients in cold climates and those who benefit from heat on their pelvic floors and low backs find heated car seats very helpful.
- **Wear a pad or guard under your clothes** if you aren't sure about restroom accessibility. Some patients wear Eversures or Wearever absorbent underwear.
- **Refer to the the Bathroom Diaries, Sitorsquat, Have2pee, wheretowee.com, and Mizpee** for public restroom locations. Some cities also offer bathroom locations.
- **Use runpee.com** to find the best time to go to the bathroom during movies.
- **Carry a MedicAlert ID** with "interstitial cystitis" engraved in it, a letter of verification from your doctor, and a bathroom-pass from the ICA or the ICN to gain access to a restroom or to the front of a line when needed. When travelling, carry a bathroom-pass, and a current letter of verification from your doctor explaining painful urgency. Don't forget to bring your prescription medicines on the plane with you if you are flying.
- **Ask your doctor to help you get a handicapped parking permit.** You may have better luck requesting a permit for

an overlapping condition, such as fibromyalgia (FMS). Your doctor should stress your disabilities, including your difficulty waiting for a parking space and/or walking a long distance with severe urgency, especially when carrying packages. Temporary permits may also be available for vacations and special events. For information call your state motor vehicle department or look online.

- **Find a drug and grocery store that can deliver** when you need help. The extra expense can be a tradeoff or prevention for days missed at work, co-pays for doctor visits and medicines.
- **Use www.stamps.com for stamps**. Post office lines can be challenging.
- **Use gas stations that will pump gas for you**.
- **Find a cleaning person to help with difficult chores** at least once a month, if possible. (Some IC patients are able to barter for services.) Often chronic pain patients who must stay at home are expected to do all of the housework!
- **If you are seeing a very busy doctor, call ahead** of your appointment to see if the doctor is running on time and find out if you can get a same-day appointment if you are in an emergency situation.
- **Always ask your doctor to write down what you don't understand**.
- **Take notes** so you don't forget important information from your doctor.
- **Contact the ICA or ICN for local support groups**, IC/BPS literature, research updates, patient support, chat rooms, and doctors' questions and answers.
- **Read books on IC/BPS and dealing with chronic illness**.
- **Refer to the Americans with Disabilities Act** (ADA) if you experience discrimination for time taken from work for treatments and medical leave, or for being turned away for a position.
- **If you can no longer work, apply for Social Security Disability**. In 2002, the Social Security Administration (SSA) announced an official **Policy Interpretation Ruling** for in-

terstitial cystitis, and instructed employees how to process disability claims for IC/BPS patients. In order to make a claim, you will need a very thorough urologist or urogynecologist who is familiar with IC/BPS to help you, although you will be required to list all of the doctors who treat your conditions. Make sure that your urologist understands the extent of your disability, including limitations in sitting, standing, walking, lifting, carrying, driving, working, and environmental sensitivities. Make a list of your current symptoms for every doctor you visit. Give one copy to the doctors and keep a copy for your personal records. Also include in that list, any problems you are experiencing that interfere with your day-to-day functioning such as riding in a car, working, housework, social activities, etc. Go over this list with your doctors and ask that it be included in your medical records. Give a copy of the list to all counselors and/or therapists you see. Keep a daily log and include how many times you void, how much sleep you miss, the activities you find challenging, the medications you take, the doctors you see, etc. It is highly important to show your limitations.

To qualify for disability you must have worked for five of the past ten years. The amount of money you have paid into social security will reflect the amount you will be rewarded, if you are rewarded. Some patients hire a lawyer or representative before they apply. Lawyers or representatives can be found through a disability advocacy group, legal aid, or through other patients. Lawyers or representatives can also help your doctor write the letter to SSDI.

Some patients try to win their claims on their own. Either way, it is best to apply for Social Security in person. You will need to present a letter from your doctor. The letter must include your diagnosis, as well as the method of diagnosis, your limitations and disabilities, especially your physical ones, how long you have had the condition and the fact that there is no cure. It should also include how many times a day you void and should focus on "why you cannot work."

Bring along your medical records and some educational articles on IC/BPS (refer to the Interstitial Cystitis Network Clinical Resources and ICA pamphlets).

Your case will be turned over to DDS (Disability Determination Services), which makes the decision on your claim. An Examiner will review your medical records and you may be sent to a doctor and/or psychiatrist for evaluation. These professionals might not understand IC/BPS or may have biased opinions about the condition. If they conclude that you are capable of performing some type of work and deny your claim, they may suggest another type of work for you. At this point, it will be necessary to find a disability lawyer for representation and perhaps contact your senator and/or congressman. The lawyer will not require payment but will be entitled to a percentage of disability payments from the time you were out of work to the time you go to court. *Refer to the ICA and the IC Network for more information and guidance.*

IC/BPS ranks in the top ten most expensive urological conditions. Insurance companies consider IC/BPS a high-risk condition. When possible, IC/BPS patients can depend on a partner for group insurance. Independent insurance is sometimes denied or the cost is too high because of a pre-existing condition.

Resources

Books

You Don't Look Sick! Living Well with Invisible Chronic Illness
Joy H. Selak, Ph.D., and Steven S. Overman, M.D., M.P.H.
www.chronicinvisibleillness.com

Chapter Eight

MANAGING SEX, MENOPAUSE, PREGNANCY, AND IC/BPS

Sex and IC/BPS

A majority of IC/BPS patients experience *dyspareunia,* which means painful intercourse. Painful sex is not exclusive to heterosexual intercourse and can be experienced with stimulation and foreplay, insertion, penetration, and/or orgasm. The most common pain in female IC/BPS patients is "thrust dyspareunia" or "deep dyspareunia." These terms are self-explanatory to female patients with dypareunia. But pain occurring during sex and/or after sex, which often sets off a pain cycle, is not exclusive to females.

When most people think about sexual activity, their thoughts turn to foreplay and intercourse that ends with orgasm. But many people with chronic pelvic pain find that sexual activity is not always that simple. Understanding the physical changes that occur during the four categories regarding the cycle of sexual response can help make sense of the problem.

The first phase of sexual response is called the desire, arousal, or the initial excitement phase. The second phase is called the plateau phase and the third, the orgasmic phase. The cycle of sexual response ends with the resolution phase.

The Excitement/Arousal Phase

During the first phase of sexual excitement or arousal, heart rate, muscle tension, and blood flow to the genitals increase. Nipples harden and become erect. The skin may flush.

Women experience swelling of their clitoris and inner vaginal lips. Vasoconstriction (caused by the massive capillary growth and numerous blood vessels) of their vaginal walls produces vaginal lubrication as the walls become tighter and smoother. The uterus rises to become more vertical and the breasts slightly swell.

Men, during the excitement phase, experience an increase in blood flow to the penis, which causes swelling and erection. Their testicles also swell and their scrotum becomes tense and thick. A secretion, that lubricates the urethra for semen to pass through, is produced by the bulbourethral glands (located in the perineal pouch). The secretion also neutralizes traces of acidic urine in the urethra.

The preparatory responses of the excitement phase are meant to make sex more comfortable. But when these responses are compromised by a particular sensitivity to vasoconstriction, and/or irritated pelvic floor muscles, or maybe even just the anticipation of pain, the brain has a difficult time releasing the pleasure-related neurotransmitters that heighten (good) sensitivity and promote relaxation and pleasure. Since the brain and the body work together during sexual activity, pain or the fear of pain may make it difficult for patients to "stay in the moment," which is necessary for physical pleasure. (The limbic system is involved in sexual desire.)

The Plateau Phase

Both females and males experience increased breathing, heart rate, blood pressure, and muscle tension during the plateau phase. Blood flow to the vagina turns the vaginal walls a dark purple color and the labia become engorged. The clitoris becomes sensitive and draws in to avoid direct stimulation. The Bartholin glands (also referred to as the greater vestibular glands) produce more lubrication. The cervix and uterus elevate, and the pubo-coccygeus muscle, the hammock-like pelvic floor muscle that extends from the pubic bone to the coccyx, the tail bone, in both sexes, tightens to reduce the opening of the vagina.

> *The Bartholin glands are located on the left and right just below the opening of the vagina and are comparable to the bulboure-thral glands in males.*

In males, the urethral sphincter contracts to prevent urine from mixing with semen. Steady contractions at the base of the penis and an increase in blood flow further swell the penis and keep it erect. Testicles draw up closer to the perineum (the space between the penis and the anus).

The Orgasmic Phase

The short orgasmic phase follows the plateau phase. When heart rate, blood pressure, and oxygen intake increase, so do involuntary muscular contractions. Orgasm in females involves contraction of the walls of the outer vagina, uterus, clitoris, ure-thra, and bladder, as well as the sphincter muscle of the rectum. Orgasm propels sperm up into the vaginal walls and into the uterus. The male orgasm is associated with muscle contractions at the base of the penis. Ejaculation involves the ducts connecting the testes, the prostate, and the penis when forcing the semen out. Ejaculation is typically felt in the penis and loins. Sensations may also be felt in the lower spine or back, but men with IC/BPS and/ or PFD may experience intense pain with orgasm and ejaculation.

The Resolution Phase

Normally, after orgasm there is a resolution phase. Blood is pumped away from the pelvis and organs relax and return to nor-mal size. Both partners experience muscular relaxation as their bodies return to the state of functioning before the excitement phase. However, IC/BPS patients can experience prolonged vaso-constriction because the nerve pathways of the bladder become involved when the irritation is stimulated during intercourse. Women may have pain and throbbing in the clitoris, bladder, urethra, and behind the vagina. Male patients may experience pain at the tip of the penis, suprapubic pain, scrotal, and/or rectal pain.

Other symptoms occurring after orgasm or sexual activity may include frequency, burning, low back, and leg pain. Because of the inflammatory condition in the bladder, and hyperactive pelvic muscles, orgasm can trigger a flare-up. Females may experience a delayed flare-up of symptoms caused by irritation of the urethra, bladder trigone, the very sensitive triangular region of the bladder, and/or vestibular glands. (Some patients only experience pain during sexual activity.) Patients who experience pain with and/or after orgasm may choose to stay detached in order to prevent orgasm; however, they may not experience the same relaxation that usually follows orgasm.

Bladder pain can result from orgasm during an erotic dream.

Pain is a signal to make one aware that something isn't working as it should. Generally, painful sex in IC/BPS patients is caused by an irritation in the bladder, but there are many IC/BPS patients who have overlapping conditions that add to painful sex. Among these is a common condition called *pelvic floor dysfunction* (PFD) (also described in Chapter One and Chapter Four). PFD is sometimes referred to as *vaginismus* in women. As mentioned earlier in the book, it's a condition which causes the pelvic floor muscles to involuntarily spasm in response to an irritant. In IC/BPS patients it seems the irritation is in the bladder. However, because the symptoms of PFD and IC/BPS are similar, doctors do not agree on whether the symptoms of IC/BPS cause the PFD, or the PFD causes IC/BPS. What most doctors do agree on is that at least 70 percent of IC/BPS patients have an abnormal cooperation of parts in their pelvic floor muscles.

Symptoms of pelvic floor dysfunction include urinary urgency and frequency, a feeling of incomplete urination, and a decreased urine flow. Urination is dependent on muscle coordination between the bladder and pelvic floor muscles. The muscles of the pelvic floor are meant to relax while the bladder contracts to urinate. However, in PFD, the pelvic floor muscles continue to tighten when the bladder contracts. This results in poor urine flow. Pushing and straining to empty the bladder further aggravates the pelvic floor muscles and creates a vicious cycle.

Pelvic floor muscles also need to be relaxed for comfortable sexual activity but they can remain tight and tense in a "guarding reflex" caused by the pain and/or urgency of IC/BPS. Sexual function, urination, and defecation are all dependent on normal contraction and expansion of the pelvic floor muscles, and PFD is associated with and/or contributes to some of the other overlapping conditions, such as chronic prostatitis.

Medical Diagnosis of Pelvic Floor Dysfunction

Although it doesn't take a doctor to tell the IC/BPS patient they have a painful condition that causes pelvic floor muscles to shorten and spasm, there is a pelvic exam to confirm a diagnosis of abnormal contraction of pelvic floor muscles. During the exam a doctor or trained physical therapist palpates the patient for pelvic floor muscle tenderness and trigger points in the vagina in a woman, or the rectum in a man. The exam includes palpation of the very tight, and usually weak and sensitive muscle in the IC/BPS patient called the pubococcygeal muscle or PC. The exam must be done very gently or it can trigger symptoms in the bladder, and referred pain in the hips, low back, and legs. Some doctors also do an uroflow test to determine urine flow, the volume of urine, and the strength of the urine stream. A probe (a type of ultrasound) is placed over the pubic bone after the patient urinates to see if there is retained urine left in the bladder.

If a diagnosis of pelvic floor dysfunction is established, a doctor can prescribe medications, such as vaginal diazepam suppositories, pelvic floor therapy sessions that also address sacroiliac (SI) dysfunction, trigger point injections to release and relax the high-tone pelvic floor muscles, and Botox injections. *Refer to Chapter Four.*

Patients should avoid denervation.

Intercourse and Pain Management

There are actually several pain management options to try before and/or after sexual activity:

- antispasmodics—Levsin (hyoscyamine), Anaspaz (hyoscyamine sulfate), Ditropan (oxybutynin) chloride
- anticholinergics—Urispas (flavoxate)
- anticholinergenics and anesthetics—Urised
- anesthetics—Pyridium, Pyridium Plus (phenazopyridine hydrocholoride)
- pain medications—opiods (*see Chapter One*)
- numbing gels—topical and vaginal lidocaine jelly, lidocaine urethral gel, amitriptyline in topical form, topical suprapubic NSAD gel or cream, Cromolyn in gel or cream for the genital area. (When numbing agents are applied in the vagina or on the penis before intercourse, a condom is needed to prevent transference of the agents.)
- anesthetic bladder instillations—lidocaine, Marcaine
- suppositories—compounded Valium or plain Valium tablets (not intended for anal use), lidocaine or Marcaine, B&O (belladonna) suppositories used after sexual activity
- Flector patches (a NSAID)
- compounded Viagra (sildenafil)—vaginal suppository or cream (Viagra appears to relieve symptoms in men with bladder and prostate problems and can sometimes be prescribed for women.)
- portable interferential stimulators
- lumbar sympathetic nerve block

Urologist Kristine Whitmore prescribes a (mild) compounded lidocaine urethral gel combined with cromolyn, a mast cell stabilizer for allergies and asthma, and a homeopathic remedy called Traumeel. Pain specialist Daniel Brookoff used urethral lidocaine gel combined with diazepam (Valium), Marcaine, or ropivacaine.

Warming or Cooling Muscles Before and/or After Intercourse

Many patients already use heat and/or cold for their flare-ups and can easily incorporate these therapies for pain prevention and management.

- **Place a warm gel pack on your pelvic floor for five to ten minutes before intercourse.** (Make sure that it is not too hot.) The warmth of a hot pack can help provide an even blood supply and relax the pelvic floor muscles. Patients who cannot tolerate the stimulation of foreplay may want to try this option.
- **Numb the vulva and vaginal tissues with cold therapy before sexual activity.** Wrap a cold pack in a thick towel and apply to the vulva for 10 to 15 minutes. A cold pack can also be used for twenty minutes after sexual activity.
- **Chill uncooked rice in a tube sock and place over the vulva.** (Make sure the tube sock is 100 percent cotton.) Premade rice packs that can be heated or chilled can be used before or after sexual activity, but scented, premade rice packs should be avoided.
- **Apply the EndoFemm.** EndoFemm is a corn-based compress that conforms to the pelvic area and can be used hot or cold.
- **Insert the Pyrex Basic Glass Wand, Bubble Glass Wand, the EZ Magic, or EZ Fit device to cool, warm, or massage vaginal and rectal muscles.** (Some patients like to warm the tissues and muscles before sexual activity and cool them after.)
- **Insert a bladder-safe condom that has been filled with water and frozen.** A frozen condom can numb the vaginal tissues before sexual activity and/or sooth irritated vaginal tissue after intercourse. The Cool Water Cone can also be used and does not require freezing.
- **Place a BodiHeat heating pad on the lower abdomen to relax the bladder after sexual activity.** The pad adheres to the outside of underwear and lasts 12 hours, but it is not intended for use while sleeping.

- **Take a hot bath or Jacuzzi before intercourse to warm and relax the whole body.** Relaxing muscles before sexual activity can help both sexes. Inviting a partner to join in may also be beneficial. Warm water not only relaxes muscles, it encourages play and sensuality. Some patients prefer a warm bath after sexual activity. Relaxing in a warm bath can reduce spasms and swelling without the friction of spot cleansing.

Applying direct heat after intercourse can increase vasoconstriction, inflammation, and the risk of infection. Drinking plenty of water after intercourse helps to dilute concentrated urine, reduce burning of tissues, and wash away bacteria that can end up in the bladder.

Proper Lubrication

Adequate lubrication is needed to protect the sensitive tissues and tight muscles caused by PFD and IC/BPS. If buying over-the-counter lubricants, patients should pick water-based ones, although there is no guarantee that all water-based lubricants will be bladder-safe. Many patients have found the following lubricants not only bladder-safe but also helpful.

- **Slippery Stuff** is available in two formulas (one is thicker) and is water soluble and odorless. It is also glycerin and paraban-free and can be used with condoms.
- **Desert Harvest Aloe Vera Personal Gel** is a chemical-free lubricant that can be used alone or with condoms. This gel may also be used as a salve for irritation and may be beneficial to patients with vulvodynia. It can be ordered from the IC Network.
- **Glycerin and Paraben Free Astroglide Liquid** is an odorless, water-based, water-soluble lubricant and vaginal moisturizer that can be used with condoms.
- **Replens** is a vaginal moisturizer that improves elasticity of the vaginal walls, relieves itching, irritation, and dyspareunia. Typically, it is used every three days to restore vaginal

pH to a premenopausal state, but can be used more often. It should be applied at least two hours before intercourse. (Replens contains glycerin and other ingredients that may be irritating to some patients.)

Pure safflower oil is another alternative for lubrication, but it's necessary to keep natural oils sterile, fresh, and refrigerated. When trying something new always be sure to use a very small amount and apply as far from the urethra as possible.

Alternative Positions for Intercourse

Our natural instincts tell us to avoid pain. Since certain sexual positions can increase pain and pressure, most IC/BPS patients figure out that if they have control of position and timing they are more willing to have intercourse.

Obviously, it is essential to find a comfortable angle for entry. Some females have their male partners enter from a low angle when using the missionary position in order not to irritate the urethra. Females who experience pain mostly in the back of their bladder walls and not in their urethras may find it more comfortable to be on top during intercourse. Susan Kellogg-Spadt, Ph.D., C.R.N.P., suggests in her ICA Update article, "Rekindle Your Sexuality," that the side-lying position might be one of the more comfortable positions for female patients. She explains, "the side-lying position encourages less vigorous thrusting and more of a gentle rocking motion."

Dr. Kellogg-Spadt notes that men may also do well with the side-lying position or they may try a standing position with their partners lying down. She also notes that men with IC/BPS may want to avoid intercourse with their partner on top. When a partner is on top, the position increases pressure on the suprapubic area. Of course, what feels comfortable depends on a patient's symptoms. Intercourse should always begin thoughtfully and slowly to help muscles gradually relax. A partner's understanding and patience can bring a couple closer.

Birth Control

Some doctors prescribe birth control pills to prevent ovulation in patients who experience flares with the hormonal changes of their menstrual cycle, but birth control pills contain progestational (progesterone) agents which are not always tolerated by IC/BPS patients. (There are some patients who are helped by birth control pills.) Plus, women in general who take birth control pills show higher rates of genital pain. Therefore taking the "pill" is not always an option for birth control. Other methods can also present problems; the pressure of a diaphragm can cause pain and patients may be susceptible to bladder (as well as vaginal) infections. Spermicides often irritate the bladder, vagina, or penis. They can also kill friendly bacteria, making both men and women more susceptible to infection. Women with IC/BPS may be more comfortable and experience fewer side effects if their partner wears a condom. (*See Proper Lubrication.*) However, both male and female IC/BPS patients should avoid pre-lubricated condoms, those that contain spermicides, and those made of latex if they experience latex sensitivity. Patients should always avoid long-lasting, time-released birth control or implanted methods of birth control.

Because preventive measures can be so challenging, IC/BPS patients need to rely on their partners to use the least irritating birth control possible. Women with IC/BPS who already have children or women who don't plan to have a family may consider asking their male partners to have a vasectomy.

Managing Overlapping Conditions That Can Interfere with Sexual Activity

Different conditions can cause painful sex. One condition is IC/BPS, but patients often have co-existing conditions, as well as adhesions and nerve damage from previous surgeries, injuries, and infections that contribute to their pain during sexual activity. Some female patients even experience an allergic reaction to their partner's semen after intercourse. Treatments and preventive measures for co-existing conditions may improve the particular condition, the possibility for more comfortable intercourse, and sometimes relieve IC/BPS symptoms. But as with any new treatment, patients must be aware of the possibility of triggering bladder symptoms.

Chronic Urinary Tract Infections

A urinary tract infection (UTI) can be set off by sexual activity. In IC/BPS patients, bacteria may come into contact with sensitive nerves between the bladder wall and lining, causing contraction of smooth muscle, burning, and frequency. Symptoms may be difficult to distinguish from the symptoms of IC/BPS. Patients who experience recurrent bladder infections often benefit from taking an antibiotic after sex as a preventive measure.

Patients who suffer with bladder infections after sex and do not use prevention may go through a very uncomfortable period of guessing, self-diagnosing, and wondering whether to call their doctors or not. Waiting can be very painful and puts too much responsibility on patients. Taking an antibiotic before urinalysis will interfere with the reading. Refrigerating a specimen will cause bacteria to multiply and interfere with the reading. IC/BPS patients who experience recurring infections after sexual activity need to plan prevention with their doctors and keep a medication on hand for pain management. Some patients may need to take a prophylactic antibiotic for prevention.

Doctors familiar with their patients' recurrent UTIs can prescribe a good antibiotic for prevention, or they may prescribe a month or two of suppressive antibiotics. Antibiotics, such as Macrobid (nitrofurantoin) or doxycycline, a member of the tetracycline antibiotics group, or minocycline, also a tetracycline which offers more anti-inflammatory effects than anti-infective effects, don't create much bacterial resistance so they are often prescribed. However, some IC/BPS patients may be sensitive to these antibiotics. Patients who are not prone to chronic bladder infections often use Leviquin for the random infection.

Pyridium, Urimax, or over-the-counter Azo-Standard or Uristat can be used for pain management until patients can get a prescribed antibiotic.

Prevention for patients with recurrent UTIs also includes washing the pelvic area with mild soap before sexual activity and drying the genitalia thoroughly after washing or bathing. Patients with recurrent infections or those with secondary conditions such as vulvodynia, or pudendal nerve damage, may do best by using a blow dryer on a cool setting instead of a towel. Hydration is also prevention. Because some patients cannot fully urinate after intercourse, they must drink plenty of water to dilute their urine. Concentrated urine can contribute to a UTI. If tolerated, blueberry juice works just like cranberry juice for the prevention of UTIs.

Yeast Infections

Yeast can inflame the vaginal lining and travel up the urethra causing irritation of the bladder. Although yeast supposedly does not thrive in an acidic atmosphere, which is thought to be maintained with regular sexual activity, the IC/BPS patient often suffers with yeast problems after sex. Contact and friction during intercourse can irritate the IC/BPS patient's vaginal tissue and result in a yeast infection. So can conventional sanitary pads. (Patients should use natural pads, such as Seventh Generation Pads or cotton GladRags.) In general, patients with urogenital pain syndromes and autoimmune conditions are more sensitive to bacteria and fungus. *For information on treatment and prevention of yeast see Chapter Five.*

If your gynecologist doesn't detect a yeast infection, and you are not convinced, ask your gynecologist to take a genital culture or a PCR test to determine the type of candida. Unusual species of yeast do exist.

Vulvodynia

Vulvodynia is a chronic condition that causes vulva discomfort and pain. This condition has also been known as pudendal neuralgia. The pudendal nerve runs through the pelvis to the vulva area near the hip bone, where it branches out into the nerves of the rectum, perineum, and clitoris. The pudendal nerve controls urination, defecation, and orgasm.

There is no known cause or cure for vulvodynia, but irritants including certain foods can worsen or trigger symptoms. Patients may experience mild to severe to disabling symptoms, which have been described as irritation, itching, burning, acid on the skin, knife-like pain, aching, throbbing, shooting pain, a tight drawing feeling, and/or a feeling of stretching or sucking-up. Skin abnormalities may appear on the outer genitals and/or there may be a thickening of the tissue under the skin, both caused by chronic neurogenic inflammation.

Also found in the bladder tissue of IC/BPS, patients with vul-vodynia have an abundance of mast cells in their vulva tissue. These mast cells release histamine which causes swelling, itch-ing, and burning. Vulvodynia patients have ten to fifteen more pain fibers in their vulvas than women without the condition.

Vulvodynia most commonly affects women between the ages of 18 and 25; however, vulvodynia is seen in young teens as well as older women. Like IC/BPS, the condition flares and responds to hormonal swings and menopause. Sixty percent of the patient population is misdiagnosed. Many of the patients also have problems with their bladders or have IC/BPS. About 50 to 85 percent of the female IC/BPS population suffers with vulvodynia.

The bladder, urethra, vagina, and vulva are all part of the uro-genital sinus. These organs begin as one small cell in the fetus. Later, when the cell divides, the different organs are created.

Vulvodynia is divided into two subtypes, vulvar vestibulitis and generalized vulvodynia:

Vulvar vestibulitis syndrome, also known as provoked vulvodynia, is experienced when pressure is applied to the vestibule, which is the tissue surrounding the vagina. Doctors who understand vulvodynia typically apply pressure with a moist Q-Tip and stretch areas along the vestibule to determine sensitivity. If the patient shows sensitivity and other conditions, including skin conditions that have been ruled out, she will most likely be diagnosed with vulvar vestibulitis syndrome.

The vestibule may not even appear inflamed but a gynecological examination, a tampon, sexual intercourse, and constipation can still cause pain and irritation. Anything that stretches or penetrates the opening of the vagina can cause symptoms. Vulvar vestibulitis may affect up to 30 percent of IC/BPS patients.

Generalized vulvodynia is not limited to the vestibule. Symptoms affect the folds of the vulva (the tissues surrounding the opening of the vagina and the urethra), the urethra, the clitoris, the perineum (the area between the vagina and rectum), and the rectum. Pain and discomfort travel to the groin area, inner thigh, and low back. Sexual intercourse, walking, and sitting for a long time, or on the wrong surface, can increase symptoms. Some patients, though, experience periods of remission.

Prevention of symptoms includes using natural and unscented personal care products, such as Seventh Generation Pads or GladRags, fragrance-free, non-irritating soap, cotton underwear (preferably organic), and proper lubrication during sexual intercourse. Avoiding tight pants, tight leggings, and pantyhose, washing underwear only with natural plant-based detergents, double or triple rinsing underwear, and rinsing the irritated skin often with plain water, mainly after urination, is also advised. Seventh Generation Baby Wipes or Natracare Intimate Wipes can also be used to soothe and moisturize irritated tissue. Many patients with vulvodynia find oatmeal compresses, and oatmeal or baking soda baths soothing. However, patients with IC/BPS are not usually candidates for other self-soothing treatments such as tea bag compresses and topical vitamin E.

The IC Network sells the Perineal Wash Bottle, Seventh Generation Baby Wipes, and Natracare Intimate Wipes. These wipes are usually also available at health food stores.

Dr. Clive Solomons, a retired professor and Director of Research at the University of Colorado Health Sciences Center, discovered several years ago that foods high in oxalate aggravated vulvodynia and patients with the condition had higher than normal levels of oxalate in their urine. Oxalate is the natural-occurring salt (needle-like crystals) of oxalate acid. It is found in leafy vegetables, whole grains, legumes, and nuts. Spinach and rhubarb contain the highest amount of oxalate. Urinary oxalate appears to go through the body very quickly, and some believe that too much concentration of the needle-like crystals in the bladder may irritate the tissue and nerves of the urethra. Following a low-oxalate diet helps many vulvodynia patients to control and limit flares. The high-oxalate foods believed to be the worst offenders are:

- beets
- beer
- all kinds of beans (including green beans)
- blackberries, blueberries, dewberries, gooseberries, raspberries, and strawberries
- black pepper (except in small amounts)
- broccoli
- celery
- chard
- citrus peel
- chocolate and cocoa
- coffee
- collards
- Concord grapes
- dandelion greens
- dried figs
- eggplant
- escarole
- green bell peppers (in large amounts)
- grits and hominy
- kale
- kamut
- kiwi
- leeks
- mustard greens
- okra
- parsley
- parships

- pecans and peanuts
- fresh red currants
- rhubarb
- rutabaga
- sardines
- sesame seeds
- spelt
- spinach
- yellow summer squash
- sweet potatoes
- swiss chard
- sour cherries
- tangerines
- tomato soups and sauces
- tea
- tofu
- turnip greens
- watercress
- wheat germ, wheat bran, and whole wheat products
- yams

IC/BPS patients with vulvodynia may obviously feel challenged when trying to eliminate another list of foods. Fortunately, IC/BPS patients and authors Bev Laumann and Julie Bayer offer information and/or recipes which are low in oxalate, as well as bladder-friendly, in their books. *The Low Oxalate Diet Book* can be ordered from the Vulvar Pain Foundation. *See Resources.*

Some patients feel caught between vulvodynia and IC/BPS, not knowing where their pain is coming from. A good urogynecologist can help patients to identify and understand their symptoms. IC/BPS patients with mild vulvodynia may find only a few of the high-oxalate foods irritating. Vulvodynia patients who are vegetarians must network with other vegetarian patients to meet their nutritional needs. Registered dieticians should be able to create friendly meals for IC/BPS and vulvodynia patients.

An additional approach to prevention of vulvodynia symptoms is taking calcium citrate supplements (without vitamin D or Polycitra). Calcium citrate is thought to help flush the oxalate out of the body by binding and neutralizing it. Although some vulvodynia patients with IC/BPS have reported that taking the supplements has helped both their bladder and vulvodynia symptoms, IC/BPS patients who are sensitive to supplements may not be able to tolerate calcium citrate.

Treatment for vulvodynia symptoms varies for both subtypes of the condition. Patients may find relief with many different types of medications, both over-the-counter and prescription. These include yeast medications (patients are vulnerable to yeast overgrowth), topical estrogen creams, and sometimes testosterone, anesthetic gels, such as lidocaine, oral pain-blocking medications, including tricyclic antidepressants, such as amitriptyline, antiseizure drugs, such as neurontin, SSNRIs, such as Cymbalta and Effexor (SSNRIs may trigger IC/BPS symptoms), opiod analgesics, Valium (diazepam) or Ativan (lorazepam) to assist sleep, anti-bacterial, anti-viral, and compounded medications, such as compounded vaginal amitrityline. Electrical stimulation, either with a vaginal probe or small pads placed on the vulva, and biofeedback may be prescribed to fatigue pelvic floor muscles. (Most IC/BPS patients cannot tolerate vaginal probes.) Sacral neuromodulation can be used for both types of vulvodynia. Nerve blocks, including pudendal nerve blocks, pelvic floor therapy, used to treat associated symptoms, trigger point injections, and Botox injections (which usually work better for vulvodynia than IC/BPS) are sometimes successful. Because of the close relationship of vulvodynia to IC/BPS, treatment for IC/BPS symptoms may help some vulvodynia patients. In severe cases of vulvodynia, inflamed tissue can be surgically removed.

Patients who are sensitive to lidocaine may try suprapubic gels, such as ketoprofen or Voltaren (diclofenac), to treat pelvic pain.

Similar to the treatments for IC/BPS, treatments for vulvodynia help some patients and not others, and/or may trigger a flare-up of symptoms. Oral medications can contain ingredients that aggravate the condition. Topical creams and ointments often contain substances, such as propylene glycol, sulfates, alcohol, and fragrance which have been known to irritate the condition of vulvodynia, as well as IC/BPS. (Creams typically contain more ingredients than ointments.)

As mentioned before, the cause of vulvodynia remains unknown but experts speculate several causes:

- an injury or irritation of the nerves that supply sensation to the vulva (including chemical irritation, certain medications, and invasive treatments)
- environmental factors, such as an infection (including viral infection) or trauma (childbirth, surgery, and invasive treatments) that cause an abnormal cellular response
- a genetic factor
- hypersensitivity to yeast

Symptoms may also relate to widespread body pain and/ or pelvic floor muscle weakness, spasm, and instability, which brings up the same question asked about IC/BPS: What comes first, the condition or pelvic floor dysfunction? What is certain, interstitial cystitis/bladder pain syndrome, vulvodynia, endometriosis, fibromyalgia, irritable bowel syndrome, migraine headaches, tempomandibular joint disorder, and multiple chemical sensitivity can co-exist. Some experts suggest that these conditions may be caused by a dysfunction in the musculature system? The Overlapping Conditions Alliance (OCA) is working hard to answer this and other questions. *Refer to Resources.*

Endometriosis

Although endometriosis can affect bladder function, the condition was not typically associated with IC/BPS until it began showing up in a number of IC/BPS patients. After seeing the overlap, Maurice K. Chung, M.D., dubbed the two conditions as "the evil twins of chronic pelvic pain syndrome." Endometriosis is now considered another inflammatory condition that can co-exist with IC/BPS.

Endometriosis is defined as a hormone and immune system disease. With endometriosis, fragments of endometrium tissue (from the lining of the uterus) travel from the uterus into the abdominal cavity where they can implant on the various pelvic organs. The fragments of tissue develop into tumors, nodules, implants, or lesions which, like the uterus, respond to the menstrual cycle by bleeding and shedding.

The fragments, growths, and lesions affect the area where they are located. When they adhere to the bladder and/or intestines, they can cause swelling and pain and interfere with elimination and urination. But fragments most commonly adhere to the ovaries, fallopian tubes, the supporting ligaments, and outer surface of the uterus, the area between the vagina and rectum, and the lining of the pelvic cavity. Growths may also be found on the rectum, female genitalia, and abdominal surgical scars. Rarely, endometrial growths are found outside of the abdomen, in the lungs and chest cavity lining, and the limbs of the body. Occasionally ovarian cysts are the result of endometriosis.

Patients with endometriosis may experience pain before and during periods, spotting, abnormal periods or heavy bleeding, pelvic and low back pain, painful intercourse and/or pain afterwards, problems with colon and bladder activity, fatigue, and infertility. Endometriosis can cause internal scarring and may increase IC/BPS symptoms, especially during sexual intercourse. When endometriosis is very severe, a hysterectomy may be needed.

A laparoscope is used to diagnose endometriosis. A biopsy is taken if endometrial tissue is not clearly recognizable. During a laparoscopy, visible endometrium tissue can be eliminated with laser or with electrocautery. Although these procedures are often helpful, they are temporary and may trigger IC/BPS symptoms during the healing process. Most doctors turn to routine treatments first, such as hormonal therapies to prevent ovulation. Birth control pills, progesterone drugs, testosterone derivative (danazol), and GnRH agonists (gonadotropin releasing hormone drugs) are usually prescribed. IC/BPS patients may experience symptoms with progestins or the progestational agents in birth control pills, and may suffer from the lack of estrogen with in-duced menopause. Complementary medicine and alternative treatments, including supplements (especially Omega 3) and ap-propriate exercise, are sometimes prescribed to patients.

Endometriosis affects females as young as eight and women after menopause. According to the Endometriosis Association, patients are at a greater risk of six cancers: ovarian and breast cancer, melanoma, non-Hodgkin's lymphoma, brain and thyroid cancer. Patients with endometriosis may also be at risk for other diseases, such as multiple sclerosis, rheumatoid arthritis, Hashi-moto's thyroiditis (which causes hypothyroidism), Sjögren's syndrome, chronic fatigue syndrome and fibromyalgia, and IC/BPS. Chemicals such as dioxin and PCBs are known to cause en-dometriosis because they mimic hormones found in the body and damage the immune system. *Refer to Chapter Six.*

Sjögren's Syndrome (Sicca Syndrome)

Some IC/BPS patients have a chronic inflammatory condition called Sjögren's syndrome. As a whole-body syndrome, Sjögren's causes white blood cells to attack the secretory glands, which leads to excessive dryness throughout the body. Thought to be an autoimmune disease, Sjögren's has no known cause and mostly affects women. Also known as sicca syndrome, a dry mouth and dry eyes are considered the hallmark symptoms of this disease. Dryness and inflammation can affect other mucous membrane linings, such as the lining of the gastrointestinal tract, trachea, vulva, and vagina. The lack of saliva in the mouth can lead to cavi-ties, difficulty swallowing, and a lack of taste and smell. Cornea damage can occur because of a lack of tears, and dry tissue in the vagina can lead to irritation, sometimes resulting in infection. Organs may also be affected in some patients.

Most women with Sjögren's syndrome are middle-aged, but Sjögren's can affect all age groups in both sexes. Symptoms of menopause usually make estrogen replacement, including topical estrogen, necessary. Proper lubrication and warming-up pelvic muscles slowly before sexual activity are recommended.

Dealing with Sex and Your Partner

Sex can enhance the quality of life, but if your last experience was painful, it's a normal reaction to avoid intercourse or even think about sex. However, it can be all too easy to let time slip by and not address sexual issues with your partner. When sexual issues aren't addressed, they can contribute to intimacy avoidance, which can lead to tension and fighting. The nature of the illness can make both you and your partner feel guilty: You, for not wanting sex, and your partner for feeling demanding or selfish when he or she knows you are in pain. Feelings can be confusing and emotional, causing communication to break down. Your partner can easily feel rejected, but so can you, even when you are the one saying *no.*

Aside from painful intercourse there may be another problem that interferes with sexual activity. Along with the symptoms of IC/BPS often comes a swollen belly and/or muscles that have gotten out-of-shape. Some patients may have a difficult time feeling desirable. Although a number of different factors go into one's self-image, self-image influences sexuality. Feeling attractive can be a challenge. This is why it is essential for IC/BPS patients to take as much control of their bodies as possible. First come IC/BPS treatment and pain prevention. Next comes control of the whole body through gentle stretching and exercise. Even if medications add body weight and negative feelings, taking a little routine exercise every day or so will help to add strength, release tension and negative feelings, and build self-esteem. Self-nurturing also includes eating healthy foods, indulging in new clothes, furniture, plants, and make-up, and/or participating in activities that promote feelings of wholeness and confidence.

Although your partner might not always show it, IC/BPS pain has an effect on him or her, too. However, a partner who chooses to ignore your pain makes it difficult for you to demonstrate affection. Natural bonding and intimacy can suffer, because everyone needs touch and care. In order to get a relationship back on track you may have to show a little spontaneity and take advantage of the times when you feel better. Although you may have difficulty being spontaneous and deserve to have your pain and needs recognized, surprising a partner with a favorite dinner, a back rub or reservations at a favorite restaurant can be very reassuring and recreate the necessary bonding that keeps relationships alive.

If a relationship has suffered, a good marriage counselor can help. A strong marriage can survive IC/BPS and IC/BPS can strengthen a good relationship. If a partner leaves a relationship and blames IC/BPS, there were probably other problems in the first place.

Having IC/BPS does not necessarily affect sexual function, but the associated pain, as well as certain medications (mainly antidepressants and opiods) and treatments, can interfere with libido and performance in both sexes. Patients who experience pain with sexual activity often become vigilant and protective, needing to keep a close watch during their sexual involvement. Although the pain that occurs with sexual activity is very real and physical in origin, emotional effects may stem from the fear of pain, the pressure to perform, and a challenged sexual identity. Patients may understandably push away their sensuality.

Sex therapist and author of *The Book of Love*, Laura Berman, Ph.D., suggests that people can rekindle their sensuality by bringing mindfulness into their daily lives: "whether it's feeling the sun on their skin or the wind on their face." This is good advice. So often, IC/BPS patients must stay mentally distracted from physical sensations because of their chronic physical pain and/or associated symptoms. Whether it's acupuncture, bodywork, and/ or pelvic floor therapy, hands-on care can usually reintroduce comfort in the body and wake up sensuality.

Dealing with Sex and a New Lover

Our youth oriented society seems to be defined by sexuality. Sex is everywhere and everyone is influenced. The younger IC/BPS patient must mature quickly, accept limitations, assume responsibility, and be realistic about who she or he is and who she or he will become. It is important for a young person with IC/BPS to be protective when first getting to know someone special. There is no need to explain problems until one is sure that the other person is sincere and mature. Having IC/BPS does not have to keep a person from being desirable or intimate. If a new partner is understanding and willing to be pro-active, helps with pain management, prepares cold packs or whatever, he or she is a team player.

IC and Younger Couples

When IC/BPS strikes the younger couple who are just beginning a life together, the effects can be quite different from those who have been together for a time. What the relationship is based on will determine how it can handle the illness. If a couple are good friends and communicative, they probably will be able to work through any sexual issues. They can develop a very strong bond, and if they choose to start a family, they can probably do so with a strong commitment.

IC, Hormones, and Mid-Life Changes in Women

IC/BPS is not considered a progressive disease. Some research has shown that the symptoms of IC/BPS reach their peak and level off after about five years, yet symptoms still can and do change with the hormonal swings in women during their menstrual cycle, during pregnancy, and during menopause. A number of female IC/BPS patients report that they experienced their first IC/BPS symptoms after having a hysterectomy. Although men with IC/BPS also experience hormonal changes that affect their prostate and bladder symptoms, their hormones stay fairly steady until they age. Because there is not yet much information available on IC/BPS, men, and hormones, this section will focus on the role of hormones in women with IC/BPS.

Research shows that hormonal changes affect systemic conditions with flare-ups and remissions, such as IC/BPS, endometriosis, fibromyalgia (FMS), chronic fatigue syndrome (CFS), vulvodynia, multiple chemical sensitivity (MCS), irritable bowel syndrome (IBS), Sjögren's syndrome, lupus (SLE), and multiple sclerosis (MS). Migraines, yeast infections, and other conditions are also triggered by hormonal swings, especially during perimenopause. Until recently, many illnesses and chronic conditions mostly prevalent in women have been blamed on psychological causes. (For example, endometriosis used to be referred to as the working woman's disease.) Also, until quite recently, hormone research has mainly been applied to male patients. However, today hormone research in women has become a big topic offering new information almost daily.

Hormonal Changes During the Menstrual Cycle

The first day of the menstrual period is also day one of the menstrual cycle. Although both estrogen and progesterone are at their lowest levels on day one, estrogen begins to rise and continues to rise after menstruation. The rise in estrogen levels thickens the uterus in preparation for fertilization. The rise in estrogen also thickens the bladder lining during this time. Estrogen levels reach their peak at ovulation, at about day 14 of the cycle.

During the first two weeks of the menstrual cycle only a small amount of progesterone is present. However, after the egg is released during ovulation, estrogen levels quickly decline and progesterone levels begin to rise in preparation for pregnancy. Although estrogen levels also begin to rise again, they stay at a lower level than that of the first half of the menstrual cycle. During this second half of the menstrual cycle, estrogen and progesterone levels reach a peak at around the same time, about the third week after the menstrual cycle. If the egg released during ovulation has been fertilized, the progesterone levels remain high. If the egg has not been fertilized, both the progesterone and estrogen production diminish quickly. The decline of progesterone levels causes the shedding of the endometrium (the uterine lining), which begins a new menstrual cycle.

IC/BPS and the Menstrual Cycle

There is no set pattern for IC/BPS patients. There are patients who experience an increase in swelling, pressure, pain, and frequency when estrogen levels are highest. This is believed to happen because estrogen increases bladder mast cell secretion, therefore increasing inflammatory reactions. During this time IC/BPS patients may help to reduce their symptoms by avoiding fermented, and hot or spicy foods that increase histamine activity.

There are IC/BPS patients who feel better when their estrogen levels are high. They experience more comfortable intercourse, can eat more varied foods with less irritation, and have more energy. Experts believe that IC/BPS patients may benefit from the increase in the thickness of the bladder lining and the lack of progesterone during this time.

Some IC/BPS patients say they feel best and experience less IC/BPS symptoms during their menstrual period when hormone levels are low. However, other patients experience bladder pain during their periods, and almost all IC/BPS patients complain of symptoms a few days prior to the onset of bleeding. A number of IC/BPS patients also report pain around ovulation when hormone levels fluctuate. Experts may disagree about the effects hormones have on the IC/BPS bladder, but what they consistently agree upon is that the bladders of IC/BPS patients react to the rise and fall of hormone levels.

> *Women in general find they have a stronger libido during their period supposedly because progesterone is at its lowest level during menses. Some experts blame progesterone for putting a damper on libido.*

IC/BPS and PMS (premenstrual syndrome)

PMS occurs during the second half of the menstrual cycle when progesterone levels are at their highest. Common symptoms include fluid retention, irritability, headaches, backache, and sometimes abdominal pain. The lower estrogen levels and high progesterone levels make some IC/BPS patients more susceptible to bladder symptoms.

> *FMS researchers have found that high levels of progesterone cause a drop in the diffuse noxious inhibitory control (DNIC) system which provides a pain-fighting function. Levels of dopamine and serotonin (the feel-good neurotransmitters) may also plunge with the drop in estrogen levels. When estrogen levels are high and progesterone levels are low, there is a greater amount of opioid activity in the pain-processing areas of the brain.*

Patients with chronic conditions may also experience fatigue, stiff muscles, abdominal pressure, and constipation when bowel activity slows down during this time. High levels of progesterone appear to worsen symptoms in women with fibromyalgia (FMS). Sensitivities to the environment and to certain drugs may also be intensified during PMS. IC/BPS patients can try to reduce bladder symptoms by following a diet for IC/BPS, avoiding salt, sugar, caffeine, increasing fiber intake, eating small meals frequently (instead of three large meals), and engaging in some form of gentle exercise.

Perimenopause and Menopause

Perimenopause, sometimes referred to as "the climacteric," begins when a woman's estrogen levels start to decline. This decline usually begins in a woman's late 30s or early 40s; however, a few women can begin to experience perimenopausal symptoms in their early 30s. The average length of perimenopause is five to ten years.

Menopause (the cessation of periods) is believed to occur between the age of 45 and 55, with the average age at 51. Menopause can happen quickly or take two to four or more years. When a woman has had no menstrual period for 12 months and blood tests confirm the decline of estrogen, menopause is considered official. A woman is no longer in perimenopause. Instead, she is now in postmenopause. A woman who has her ovaries removed with hysterectomy has what is called surgical menopause.

Symptoms During Perimenopause

Symptoms vary woman to woman because the approach to menopause is so individual. Fluctuations of estrogen create hormonal swings which in turn can cause night sweats, waking episodes, insomnia, hot flashes, chills, palpitations, lighter, heavier, or irregular periods, complexion problems, depression, and troubles with memory and concentration. Women in early perimenopause can experience lighter periods, night sweats, insomnia, painful PMS, and constipation. As hormone levels continue to drop, symptoms can change. Blood tests are used to determine hormone levels.

Physical Changes that Affect the Bladder During Perimenopause

All women experience change in their bladders and vaginas during menopause. Estrogen directly affects the bladder lining, nerves, blood vessels, and muscles that control urinary function. When estrogen levels begin to decline, the smooth muscle in the bladder, urethra, and vagina loses tone and strength. This decline in estrogen concurrently increases sensitivity to pain and susceptibility to bladder problems.

As estrogen levels decline, so do levels of serotonin, which is a pain fighter.

When there is a decrease in blood flow and lubrication, the urethral, bladder and vaginal tissue becomes thinner, drier, less resilient, and more susceptible to inflammation. Supporting muscles and tissue of the bladder and uterus lose tone and stability, allowing the bladder to fall downward. The dropping of the bladder can change the angle of the urethra, making the bladder more susceptible to outside bacteria. These various changes leave the bladder vulnerable to infection and can cause symptoms such as urgency, frequency, burning, and sometimes mild incontinence (IC/BPS does not lead to or cause incontinence). Women who suffer with chronic urethral pressure, frequency, and other bladder symptoms may be diagnosed with urethral syndrome. Urethral syndrome is sometimes treated with bladder dilation. Dilation should be avoided because it can cause scarring, injury, and incontinence, as well as worsen the symptoms of IC/BPS, even if IC/BPS is experienced later.

As IC/BPS patients begin to reach menopause, their IC/BPS symptoms can also change. Patients who are used to feeling relief upon urination (due to the lack of blood flow when voiding) may experience some burning in their urethras instead. Patients in early perimenopause may begin to notice cramping in their pelvic floor around ovulation, right before or after their menstrual period. Patients who also have endometriosis or IBS may experience more pain from inflammation and built-up scar tissue as hormones begin to decline. In general, women with injured muscles and ligaments from surgeries, childbirth, or low back problems may experience compounded weakness and bladder problems. Pressure on pelvic veins can cause painful varicose veins, pelvic and leg pain. Perimenopause is a time to keep back muscles strong, use good support while sitting, and avoid lifting heavy objects.

Coping with IC/BPS and Other Conditions During Perimenopause

Many patients are in perimenopause when diagnosed with IC/BPS. It's easy to comprehend the challenge of a chronic condition during perimenopause. Symptoms such as disturbed sleep, palpitations, constipation, fatigue, muscle pain, and weakness are often intensified at this time. Determining which symptoms are part of perimenopause and which are part of the chronic illness may be difficult and confusing. However, symptoms should not be ignored. Women in general must begin to listen to their bodies more closely, and IC/BPS patients may need to be aware of common overlapping conditions that may occur during perimenopause.

Heart palpitations may be a natural symptom of perimenopause and may sometimes be uncomfortable for IC/BPS patients with mitral valve prolapse (MVP). However, palpitations can also indicate a heart condition or more often in IC/BPS patients, a thyroid disorder. Thyroid production decreases as one ages and women who experience irregular and run-away periods, fatigue, heart palpitations, and anxiety attacks, as well as painful PMS, should ask their doctors for thyroid screening, including free T3 and T4 levels. This screening should be done along with hormone levels tested during perimenopause, because it is not unusual for IC/BPS and FMS patients to also have hypothyroidism, low functioning thyroid. Plus, the symptoms of hypothyroidism can be confused with the symptoms of perimenopause.

If thyroid levels turn out to be borderline and doctors do not want to prescribe thyroid medication, IC/BPS patients should ask for a repeat test. If there is no change and patients cannot get treatment for symptoms, it's time to see other doctors. Patients with chronic illnesses who test borderline, or close to, often need treatment even if the doctor does not agree. Patients with irregular periods who are given birth control pills as treatment should be aware that they can aggravate bladder symptoms in some patients.

IC/BPS patients who suffer with fatigue and shakiness may also want to ask to be tested for anemia and/or pernicious anemia (B-12 deficiency). B-12 deficiency appears to affect patients with chronic conditions and people as they age.

Vitamin B-12 is found in meat, eggs, and milk. Patients should avoid putting these foods in the microwave because microwaving is thought to inactivate the B-12.

Inflammations and infections in the vagina and bladder that occur with hormone changes are more difficult to treat for patients with IC/BPS, vulvodynia, Sjögren's syndrome, CFS, IBS, and patients with chronic yeast infections. Natural fatigue during perimenopause can be more challenging. Patients with migraine headaches, drug, and environmental sensitivities may also become more vulnerable to their symptoms.

It's obvious that a woman with a chronic illness feels less in control during perimenopause. The IC/BPS patient used to predicting and understanding her symptoms by her menstrual cycle will have to readjust. Menopause can be very stressful. The IC/BPS patient may have to work more closely with her urologist or gynecologist or find a urogynecologist. Estrogen replacement and/or new treatments and medications may be needed to control symptoms. It's important to realize that when periods start up, become somewhat regular, then stop again, new symptoms of IC/BPS that may accompany perimenopause can also change. Some do get better or even go away. The experience of menopause is not a final sentence. It's a time when the healthy peers of an IC/BPS patient also must slow down and pay attention to their bodies.

Hormone Replacement Therapy (HRT)

For years HRT was routinely prescribed to postmenopausal women to relieve menopausal symptoms and protect them from certain diseases. The gold standard of HRT was either Prempro, estrogen opposed with progestin (synthetic progesterone), or Premarin (estrogen only) for women who had their uterus removed. Both medications contain estrogen derived from mare's urine. Estrogen was believed to offer many benefits, such as keeping bones strong, controlling cholesterol levels, keeping arteries clear, and skin healthy and youthful. Estrogen was also thought to assist memory and concentration and perhaps help to reduce the risk of Alzheimer's disease and colon cancer. But in the mid-2000s, the results of the Women's Health Initiative Study (WHI), a study designed to evaluate the risks, benefits, and disease prevention of HRT, changed most of the earlier beliefs that supported the benefits of HRT. WHI discovered that HRT could be dangerous. Clinical studies found HRT increased the risks of breast cancer, stroke, blood clots, as well as other problems, and that HRT did not improve memory and concentration.

Although the study found that HRT reduced the risks for fractures and perhaps colon cancer too, doctors stopped prescribing HRT and patients stopped taking their hormones. Today, after more studies, researchers believe it was only the estrogen in the HRT that helped to reduce fractures and possibly prevent colon cancer. And that it was really the age when women began hormone therapy that determined the benefits and risks. For example, if a woman begins HRT long after she began menopause she is at risk for heart disease and a woman who restarts HRT after a long period of time may also be at risk. On the other hand, younger women who go on HRT within ten years of beginning menopause, have less heart disease and less fatality from other causes. (The WHI did not study women in their 40s and 50s, so the other studies were necessary.)

Women taking estrogen-alone (without progestin) showed less risk for coronary heart disease. Therefore some experts believe that taking estrogen alone, for about two to three years, may be all right; however, there can be an increased risk for stroke in older women. With opposed estrogen (combination therapy) there is still a high risk for breast cancer, which may be due to progestin because estrogen-alone does not pose the same risk when taken short-term. Down the road, taking only estrogen, there may be an increased risk.

Small doses of estrogen-alone, or estrogen replacement therapy (ERT), play a role in the management of some chronic conditions. Even though estrogen is known to enhance inflammation in general, estrogen does increase elasticity of the bladder and urethra, thicken the bladder lining, and relieve bladder hypersensitivity after menopause. Many IC/BPS patients avoid severe bladder, muscle and joint pain, and constipation-IBS symptoms with estrogen replacement.

But researchers conclude that HRT (combined hormones) doesn't prevent certain diseases as they once thought it did and suggest that women take the lowest dose of HRT for the shortest period of time possible after menopause. Unlike the years before the WHI study, HRT or ERT (estrogen-alone) is now prescribed on an individual-based case.

Hormone replacement therapy is also referred to as menopausal hormone therapy (MHT).

Hormone Replacement Choices

There are standard blood tests to determine hormone levels and the appropriate dose of hormone replacement, but finding the right time to begin replacement and the correct level or type of hormone replacement is often "trial by error" for patients with IC/BPS. Patients need to work with gynecologists, urogynecologists, or naturopaths who specialize in alternative medication, to regulate hormonal balance, because everything changes during menopause, including IC/BPS.

The doctor a woman sees can determine her hormone replacement therapy. It may be a challenge for menopausal patients, who still have their uteri, to get prescriptions for estrogen-alone hormones due to the risk of uterine cancer. Because estrogen increases the risk of cell build up in the lining of the uterus, as well as other areas, a woman is usually prescribed estrogen opposed with progesterone. But doctors may not realize the full impact of hormones in IC/BPS patients. Doctors may not be aware that there are patients who cannot tolerate estrogen opposed with progesterone, but usually will understand if their patients explain that progesterone increases symptoms in women with other conditions, such as migraine headaches. If patients find understanding doctors who will prescribe a small amount of unopposed estrogen to relieve menopausal and/or bladder symptoms, the doctors will most likely suggest a routine ultrasound of the uterus and/or an endometrial biopsy whether patients experience bleeding or not. Of course, doctors must evaluate a personal health profile, as well as family history, before prescribing HRT or ERT.

The most active form of estrogen, estradiol (the estrogen routinely prescribed), is capable of causing growth of the uterus and breasts, as well as vaginal and other estrogen-sensitive tissues, such as the bladder (in which the estrogen may help by increasing the thickness of the bladder lining).

Today there is a conflict of opinions about the symptoms and benefits of progesterone. Many of those who promote natural plant progesterone blame the imbalance of progesterone and estrogen during perimenopause as the cause of PMS and menopausal symptoms. According to this belief, during menopause progesterone production can become irregular and leave estrogen unopposed. The unopposed estrogen is then believed to cause the symptoms of PMS (during perimenopause), hot flashes, bloating, insomnia, depression, and irregular periods. Some supporters of this theory believe that even the phytoestrogens in your diet must be balanced. Alternative doctors and naturopaths usually promote natural progesterone, but they also may vary in their theories and treatments.

The other school of thought (which usually consists of doctors who practice traditional medicine) is that progesterone is the cause of PMS, bloating, constipation, insomnia, headaches,

and depression. Hot flashes and irregular periods are blamed on
the decline of estrogen during perimenopause, and progestins
(synthetic progesterone) taken to oppose estrogen during HRT
(hormone replacement therapy) are blamed as the cause of constipation and bloating.

As always, what works depends on the individual IC/BPS
patient. There are some patients who cannot tolerate estrogen
or progesterone replacement. And there are patients who benefit from plant supplements. The following information reviews
some of the available hormone replacement choices. Each IC/BPS
patient must make an informed decision based on her symptoms
and the advice of a trusted doctor. It's helpful to read as much as
possible and stay abreast of new forms of hormone replacement
and new IC/BPS treatments.

Progesterone Choices

Progestogens include synthetic progestins and natural progesterone. Natural or bio-identical progesterone is derived from
plants, soy and wild yams, and exactly duplicates the progesterone that the body produces. Natural progesterone is available in
several different forms: lotions, gels, spray, patches, sublingual
drops, and vaginal suppositories. Oral progesterone acts differently than other forms of the hormone. Instead of going directly
into the bloodstream, it must first go to the liver. Both natural
progesterone and progestins produce a similar anti-growth factor
in the uterus like that of the body's own progesterone. Traditional
doctors have been skeptical about the effectiveness of natural
progesterone. They either consider it too weak and unpredictable
to treat menopausal symptoms and prevent health risks, or too
strong for unregulated, self-medication.

Doctors or naturopaths who promote natural progesterone
support the theory that it doesn't provoke the side effects of synthetic progestins, such as headaches, bloating, and weight gain.
Also, they find that unlike progestin, natural progesterone does
not interfere as severely with the benefits of estrogen.

Progestogens in general seem to be poorly tolerated by a
number of IC/BPS patients. Natural progesterones are known to
increase urinary frequency as they act as a diuretic. Progestogens

are available in tablets, capsules, vaginal suppositories, injections, creams, vaginal gels, as well as subdermal pellets which are rarely used in the U.S. Natural progesterone in cream and gel form can be found in many health food stores.

Remember, when trying vaginal creams and gels, always apply a small amount of the product as far away as you can from the urethra. Always avoid long-lasting forms of hormones. When trying an injection always ask for the smallest amount. Tell your doctor that this is an experimental dose. Otherwise you may have a long flare-up if the hormone affects your bladder.

Estrogen Choices

The available various estrogens work differently and offer different benefits. Estradiol is usually a doctor's choice of estrogen replacement for women beginning hormone replacement therapy. It is the predominant natural human estrogen most abundantly produced by the ovaries before menopause. Estradiol is also the form of estrogen that occurs naturally in plants.

There are several choices and many ways to use estrogen replacement: vaginal or topical cream, oral medication, skin patch, injection, vaginal suppositories, and internal rings (which may cause too much pressure on the pelvic floor and bladder). Many doctors now prescribe FDA approved plant-sourced estrogens. Phytoestrogens (plant estrogens) are not only available in prescription drugs, they are also prescribed by alternative doctors who promote bioidentical hormones. Some formulations are found at drug and health food stores. (Natural and bioidentical hormones are not FDA approved.) Phytoestrogens are delivered in transdermal patches, pills, and creams. Prescription estrogen creams and bioidentical hormones are processed by specialized compounding pharmacies.

Most IC/BPS patients should be given estrogen immediately after their ovaries are removed during hysterectomy. The drop in estrogen can shock the body and cause a bladder flare-up. Of course, there are some patients who cannot tolerate estrogen replacement (ERT).

Estrogen Cream Some IC/BPS patients control the early symptoms of menopause with estrogen cream which can be applied topically on the belly, thighs, vulva, or inserted vaginally. The effects of the different estrogen creams are very individual, but in general they appear not to deliver the consistent dose or systemic benefits of other forms of estrogen. This can be both good and bad, depending on the patient's needs, age, and risks factors.

The effectiveness of estrogen creams inserted vaginally also depends on the condition of the vaginal lining and thickness of the vaginal wall. Evidence so far shows that estrogen creams help to alleviate some vulvar and vaginal symptoms, such as dryness, itching, and burning with urination, and may help to prevent bladder infections. However, creams applied close to the uterus have in some instances stimulated endometrial proliferation. (All estrogen can present a risk.)

There are patients who use estrogen creams during perimenopause until they may need a stronger estrogen. Some patients continue to use a little estrogen cream topically for vulvar and urethral symptoms after they begin a stronger estrogen. Estrogen cream alone does not appear to help very much with IC/BPS symptoms, but does appear to help some women prevent certain vulvar and urethral symptoms.

Estrogen creams in general contain inactive ingredients that may irritate the bladder, urethra, and the vulva. Patients complain of reactions to propylene glycol, alcohol, and fragrance. Working with a compounding pharmacy can help patients to avoid irritating additives. Networking with other patients can also help to find a good compounding pharmacy.

Oral Estrogen Prescription oral estrogen can be animal or plant based. Patients who also have IBS may find that they do not get the consistent full benefit of oral estrogen because of poor bowel absorption. IC/BPS patients may also experience bladder pain and other reactions to the dyes and inactive ingredients in the different brands of oral estrogen, or to particular estrogens. Some women have reported muscle spasms and leg cramping thought to be triggered by equine estrogen (pregnant mares' urine) which is used in Premarin.

Since medications are very challenging, the IC/BPS patient should begin with a low level estrogen at first. This is important unless there is severe bladder pain due to the lack of estrogen. In this case a strong dosage is usually necessary. The patient may have to switch brands if the first type of estrogen isn't agreeable or does not relieve her bladder symptoms. Also, if estrogen replacement is started before needed, the IC/BPS patient can experience a negative reaction.

Estrogen Patch Many IC/BPS patients prefer to use an estrogen patch. There is less hormone needed with a patch because the estrogen and inactive ingredients do not have to be broken down in the stomach and intestines as oral estrogen does. Instead they flow through the skin into the bloodstream. Patches can contain acrylic and silicone adhesives, membranes, gels, and protective films that may be irritating to patients with sensitive skin, chemical sensitivities, and allergies. Estrogen and added ingredients in estrogen patches may also irritate the bladder. Estrogen replacement is always individual. Women who cannot tolerate estrogen replacement will usually know right away with symptoms of nervousness, headache, increased pelvic pressure, bladder discomfort, or pain.

Plant Estrogens Prescription phytoestrogens contain components that are chemically synthesized from plant material, such as soy. These compounds are similar to the estrogens found in the body. Estrogen supplements are derived from dietary and herbal sources found in soy, flax, dong quoi, and black cohosh. Prescription phytoestrogens present the same health risks as Premarin.

Slow Release Estrogen Most IC/BPS patients should avoid hormone implants and injections. Long lasting forms of slow release hormones cannot offer the same control and pain management of other forms of estrogen. Also, devices such as the estrogen ring, which is inserted like a diaphragm and about the same size, are usually not comfortable for IC/BPS patients. The benefit of the estrogen ring is that it treats vaginal symptoms and maybe bladder symptoms without the same systemic effects of other methods.

Balancing the Body with Bioidentical Hormones

Bioidentical hormones are made from yams and soy. The effects of bioidentical hormone replacement therapy (BHRT) are considered more physiologic than therapeutic. Rather than just treating the symptoms of menopause, promoters of BHRT believe it restores low levels of hormones and boosts immune responses in the body. Many researchers believe that BHRT are essential for age management and do not carry the risks of conventional synthetic hormones.

BHRT are prescribed after specific blood testing for adrenal, thyroid, and reproductive hormones. Doctors who prescribe BHRT say that restoring hormones to their normal values leads to more energy and endurance, as well as improvement in an overall sense of well-being. Randy Birken, M.D., Clinical Assistant Professor Baylor College of Medicine Fellow, American College of Obstetricians and Gynecologist Fellow, American College of Surgeons, believes that women need estrogen and progesterone, as well as testosterone, because all three hormones work synergistically (together). According to Birken, they protect against heart disease and improve bone and muscle mass. He has found that restoring his patients' levels of testosterone leads to better skin tone, more energy, and improved mood and libido.

Birken also uses compounded bio-identical thyroid to treat hypothyroidism, and he actually prescribes thyroid to patients who need a "little boost." Patients with low levels of DHEA, which is made by the adrenal glands and is precursor for all hormones, experience improved metabolism, enhanced mood, and lower cholesterol levels (due to a breakdown of fat) when taking compounded DHEA.

Dr. Birken looks at both T4 and T3 to determine if T3 is low. Low T3 can lead to a slow metabolism, fatigue, and sometimes a foggy memory. Years ago it wasn't unusual for doctors to prescribe thyroid to patients who were feeling the symptoms of hypothyroidism but tested normal.

To find physicians who understand and prescribe BHRT refer to the American Academy for Anti-Aging Medicine website. Although BHRT are not routinely covered by insurance, lab work may be coded in such a way for coverage and some compounding pharmacies will file with insurance.

Menopause Management Without Hormone Replacement

IC/BPS patients who cannot take estrogen must supplement their diet with calcium rich foods and some form of weight bearing exercise such as walking or strengthening with small weights. Those who can, should take vitamin D and eat foods for their mineral, vitamin, and estrogen properties. If patients can tolerate soy products and/or flaxseed oil, they may benefit by adding these dietary estrogens to their diet. Foods and oils that do not agree with IC/BPS patients when first tried should be avoided.

Patients with whole body symptoms may lift light weights while lying on their backs for the best support.

Vaginal dryness must be addressed to prevent inflammation and infection. Lubricants can help with prevention (*see Lubrication Choices in this chapter*) and some patients can use hydrocortisone creams to calm inflammation. However, hydrocortisone can be irritating to the bladder and should be tried very sparingly. IC/BPS patients who cannot tolerate estrogen and experience a worsening of symptoms with menopause may have to try new lubricants and medications or follow a stricter diet to calm the bladder during and after menopause. Of course, there are women with IC/BPS who feel better after perimenopause with no hormone replacement.

Postmenopause

Until recently, how long women took estrogen depended on their symptoms and what doctors were taught in medical school. Some women took hormone replacement therapy (HRT) on a regular basis for the rest of their lives. Some took HRT for two to five years after menopause. Others only took estrogen for a few months to control symptoms, and some women didn't take estrogen at all. Women who took estrogen were often advised to reduce their dosage after they had taken estrogen for a certain length of time. This was because it did not seem to be necessary and because of the increased risks of breast cancer after five to ten years. For some IC/BPS and other patients with chronic conditions, estrogen replacement may be needed for a long period of time. Today, the connection between breast cancer and estrogen (as well as other diseases) is well known and taking estrogen replacement for a long period of time is not encouraged.

Hormone replacement is serious business. Hormones are very powerful. If IC/BPS patients decide to reduce their dosage, they should taper off slowly and perhaps alternate the higher dose (the present dose) with the lower dose every other day. If women in general want to end their hormone therapy, they too should taper off slowly. This is best done with a doctor's direction and the awareness that IC/BPS patients should make changes very slowly. (Some antidepressants are used to treat menopausal symptoms but may not be bladder-friendly for IC/BPS patients. Acupuncture may be an effective treatment for hot flashes.)

Health Risks at Mid-Life

Doctors make evaluations at menopause and mid-life for both female and male patients. Tests and prevention for diseases that may present at mid-life are becoming standardized. Middle-aged patients fall into a type of "package treatment program" with insurance companies and doctors. Although IC/BPS does not exclude patients from their mid-life regime of tests and maintenance, there seems to be an excess in testing for women.

The IC/BPS patient can work best with doctors who understand and work with individual sensitivities to medicines, dyes, and liquids used during certain tests. Referred specialists and technicians who evaluate and give tests may not know or understand IC/BPS. Therefore, it's important to stay informed. *Harvard*

Women's Health Watch (health.harvard.edu/newsletters) offers current information on women's health, tests, and procedures.

Pregnancy and IC/BPS

Hormones During Pregnancy

Estrogen, progesterone, and prolactin, as well as hormones produced by the thyroid and adrenals, are active during pregnancy. In the beginning of the first trimester, progesterone levels increase quickly to prepare the uterus for pregnancy. A hormone called human chorionic gonadotropin (hCG) also increases quickly and is thought to be responsible for the ovarian production of progesterone until the end of the first trimester when the placenta takes over the production. Levels of progesterone are 30 to 50 times higher during pregnancy, than normal. Three estrogens, estradiol, estriol, and estrone, are also involved in pregnancy. Estradiol increases about 100 percent although estriol is actually considered the major source of estrogen during pregnancy. Estrone remains the least abundant estrogen.

The growth factors associated with IC/BPS are influenced by both estrogen and progesterone. Refer to Chapter One.

Bladder Changes during Pregnancy

Many patients report that they experience less bladder, muscle, and joint pain than before pregnancy. A number of IC/BPS patients go into remission. Some experts believe that remission of symptoms during pregnancy occurs in many chronic pain patients because the immune system is suppressed during pregnancy. (Female hormones regulate the immune processes in women.) Yet bladder frequency and some of the other IC/BPS symptoms are a part of pregnancy. This is especially true during the early and late part of pregnancy when there is extra pressure on the bladder. The baby drops lower in the belly in the third trimester, and hormones loosen the ligaments that hold the pubic bone parts together. Isa Herrera, M.S.P.T., C.S.C.S., clinical director of Renew Physical Therapy in New York City, suggests that patients wear a pregnancy belt to lift the belly and take the pressure off the bladder.

IC/BPS patients who also have FMS may experience a worsening of their muscle symptoms during the last trimester. IC/BPS patients in general might experience the most relief during the middle trimester.

Physically, younger women may have an easier time with pregnancy. However, many IC/BPS patients, both young and older, find they feel better than usual when they are pregnant. But a good pregnancy depends on factors other than feeling physically well. Patients need the support and understanding of others, doctors who will listen, and if needed, the guidance of family counselors.

Preparing for Pregnancy and IC/BPS

Every woman's goal is to have a healthy baby, but a woman with IC/BPS has the added goal of keeping her bladder symptoms under control during pregnancy. She quickly learns the key to success with IC/BPS and pregnancy is good planning.

A small study on IC/BPS and pregnancy showed that patients had no more problems getting pregnant than women without IC/BPS. Mothers with IC/BPS were also found to have the same rate of deliveries and healthy babies as other women.

Planning before conception may allow the IC/BPS patient to get her symptoms under control before becoming pregnant. Learning alternative pain management for symptoms before conception is beneficial throughout pregnancy because bladder treatments and medicines should typically be discontinued. Pain management before conception may mean avoiding intercourse, except, of course, during ovulation.

Pain prevention and planning are not limited to preconception. IC/BPS management is helpful throughout pregnancy, delivery, and child care, and can begin when the IC/BPS patient learns she is pregnant.

Excellent and thorough insights on pregnancy can be found in the "Pregnancy Diaries" on the ICN. Look for both "Lesa's Pregnancy and IC Diary," and "Melanie's Pre-pregnancy Check List." Referring to the information offered by the ICN and ICA can help a patient to begin her journey of pregnancy. Networking with other IC/BPS patients can also be very helpful.

Picking the Right Doctor

A woman with IC/BPS may not qualify for special, or what is called *high-risk* treatment, even when she does not comfortably fit into the routine approach. If a patient has developed a good relationship with her OB/GYN concerning IC/BPS, she may do best continuing with this doctor or she may find an OB who has experience delivering patients with IC/BPS and/or vulvodynia, and an OB who doesn't do unnecessary vaginal exams or trans-vaginal ultrasounds. However, if the IC/BPS patient feels that she may need medication during pregnancy or be intensely man-aged, the ICA has suggested that a patient consider choosing an obstetrician who specializes in high-risk pregnancy or urology. Of course, the woman with IC/BPS may still have to convince a new doctor of her unique needs. Even high-risk practitioners may not know much about IC/BPS. Sometimes a pain specialist is needed.

The IC/BPS patient may also want to ask for a thyroid function test along with her pregnancy test. The thyroid is directly linked with reproduction, and hypothyroidism (thyroid deficiency) can interfere with conception and make pregnancy more difficult. It can take a repeat thyroid test to detect low thyroid levels. If you have trouble conceiving, you may have to be persistent if you suspect that you have a thyroid deficiency.

If a fertility specialist is needed, you will most probably be treated as other women without IC/BPS. Although you have to let your doctor know that bladder pain management is a concern for you, the specialist might not be open or able to help you avoid some discomfort during fertility treatment, which may include taking hormones and certain irritating medications.

Pain Management During Pregnancy

As with the individual symptoms of each IC/BPS patient, every IC/BPS pregnancy is unique. Even though the IC/BPS patient is usually familiar with her own pain triggers, pregnancy is a time to follow stricter guidelines for IC/BPS pain prevention and to avoid most prescription treatments or medications.

Options for pain management include acupuncture (which has also been shown to help with morning sickness) and pelvic floor therapy. However, a patient's OB must be consulted first. Also, most physical therapists prefer to reserve pelvic floor therapy for the second trimester only, when there is less risk. Other options include a diet for IC/BPS, relaxation techniques, warm baths, gentle exercise, massage therapy (only with a doctor's consent), and keeping to a routine daily schedule. The bladder is calmer when the IC/BPS patient feels in control and less stressed.

Medications During Pregnancy

Dealing with your bladder can be your biggest concern besides your baby; however, at times there may be other minor conditions to deal with. You may be used to avoiding a variety of medications due to bladder sensitivity and you may use alternative treatments for minor illnesses and conditions, but during pregnancy it's necessary to work with the doctor to treat problems that arise. Self-medication, including some over-the-counter medications, should be avoided.

Even if a doctor prescribes a drug or an over-the-counter medication, it's a good idea to investigate the risks of all medications to avoid bladder pain, other sensitivities, and of course, risks to the baby's health. It is also vital to make the doctor aware of every medication that you are taking or condition you are being treated for.

Some medications or treatments are safer than others, but are usually not advised during the first trimester. In 2007 Deborah Erickson, M.D., and Kathleen Propert, Sc.D., classified the safety and risks of certain medications taken during pregnancy in their article "Pregnancy and IC/BPS," printed in Urologic

Clinics of North America. *Elmiron, amitriptyline, hydroxyzine, DMSO, sacral nerve stimulation, and some instillations were evaluated. Out of these medications and treatments, Elmiron received the highest rating of the medications. However, it was only rated as a category B drug and most doctors would prefer that their patients not take Elmiron while pregnant. Amitriptyline was considered as a "low-risk" treatment, but hydroxyzine not so safe and should be avoided because it may cause birth defects. The authors suggested that patients who use lidocaine instillations only use **non-alkalinized** lidocaine and not alkalinized lidocaine during pregnancy. Heparin instillations may also be all right, but not DMSO instillations as they have not been studied in pregnant patients. Patients with internal sacral stimulators are advised to have them turned off because there is not enough known about the effects on a fetus. The Interstitial Cystitis Network also warns pregnant patients to absolutely avoid Cytotec. In all, patients who take medications during pregnancy are considered high-risk and should consult with a high-risk pregnancy specialist. Patients who take opioids (except for methadone which usually must be avoided) have to work closely with their doctors and expect a long hospital stay for their babies after delivery. Sadly, their babies must go through detoxification.*

Diet and Pregnancy

Some IC/BPS patients experience bladder relief during pregnancy and find they can eat a greater variety of foods than before pregnancy. However, patients should be aware that food tolerance can change with the hormonal changes of each trimester. Some patients need to be more disciplined during their third trimester and some must stick to a bladder-safe diet throughout pregnancy.

Nutrition and Prenatal Vitamins

Pregnant women are advised to take prenatal vitamins and eat nutrient-rich produce high in vitamins. Tolerating the food sources and vitamins that supply the needed nutrition during pregnancy can be a challenge for IC/BPS patients. Prenatal vitamins contain lots of vitamin C and B-6 which may trigger IC/BPS symptoms. Bev Laumann suggests a helpful strategy: Pregnant IC/BPS patients can write down the amounts of each vitamin listed on their prenatal vitamin bottles. Then they can buy the individual vitamins in the listed dosages. Naturally, patients should try one supplement at a time to detect tolerance. Some patients find they can tolerate a buffered C (with calcium carbonate) or the version called "ester C." Vitamin B-12 and folate (which is a B vitamin) may be bladder-safe.

> *Because a lot of prenatal vitamins have a high amount of ascorbic acid (vitamin C), a patient may want to try children's vitamins which use sodium ascorbate instead. Some patients do well with Flintstones and find they can supplement them with additional folic acid.*

It's very important for IC/BPS patients to read up on nutrition and pregnancy. It's also necessary for patients to put a lot of color and different foods into their daily diet in order to get necessary vitamins and minerals. Some experts suggest that IC/BPS patients consult a nutritionist when there's uncertainty about meeting nutritional requirements. Understanding professionals may help patients to problem-solve, feel more supported, and less worried which is best for mom and baby. *For information on alternative vitamin sources refer to the vitamin-rich foods suggested in Chapter Two and to the following information.*

Calcium Adequate calcium is necessary during pregnancy. The IC/BPS patient who cannot tolerate calcium supplements must add extra calcium-rich foods, such as dairy products, to her diet. If dairy products are tolerable, the IC/BPS patient can drink milk and eat fresh cheeses (*refer to Chapter Two*), such as ricotta cheese (check for added vinegar), cottage cheese, cream cheese, and ice cream (the less additives in ice cream the better). Individuals with lactose intolerance can usually tolerate yogurt, which is a good source of calcium. Plain, vanilla, maple, or honey are usually best, because yogurt made with fruit contains more sugar and the fruit may be a bladder irritant.

Whole milk dairy products provide a better source of calcium than skim or low fat dairy products, because fat enhances calcium absorption. If a pregnant woman is restricted to low fat dairy products, she should eat her main source of daily calcium along with another food that contains fat. For example, she can have a glass of low fat milk with a piece of buttered toast, or with a salad dressed in olive oil or another oil-based dressing. A salad with a plain yogurt and oil dressing is also a good source of calcium and tasty with a little added fresh dill.

Other rich sources of calcium can be found in salmon, almonds, and tofu, if tolerated. (Farmed salmon should be avoided depending on the food the salmon are fed. Patients should consult with their doctors before consuming fish.) It's important to avoid foods like spinach and other dark greens when eating your main calcium source. Although these foods do offer a good source of iron and actually calcium and other nutrients, they can decrease the calcium absorption of other foods. Eating too much fiber while consuming a main source of calcium can also rob the body of needed calcium.

Iron Foods and supplements rich in iron are very important during pregnancy. Unfortunately, not all IC/BPS patients can tolerate iron supplements and therefore need to eat foods that supply a good source of iron, such as beef and other meats, poultry, fish, egg yolks, and kidney and baked beans (preferably not in tomato sauce). Nuts, if tolerated, also provide a source of iron and other minerals. Just a small handful of nuts can supply patients with a lot of nutrition. Some IC/BPS patients say that they can eat cashews, pine nuts, and almonds. Other patients can tolerate hazel, Brazil nuts, pecans, and peanuts. Patients can also make their own trail mix. Tolerated nuts can be mixed with golden raisins (without sulfates) and/or carob chips. Carob covered almonds are another good source of iron and fiber.

Iron is more easily absorbed when eaten with foods that are rich in vitamin C. Most patients cannot tolerate orange juice and other citrus fruits. However, they can eat potatoes and other produce rich in vitamin C along with meat, poultry, and fish which are the best absorbed sources of iron. *Refer to Chapter Two for produce rich in vitamin C.*

Adequate fiber is very important during pregnancy, especially when taking iron supplements which can provoke constipation. There are different iron supplements available for those who have this problem. There are also alternative supplements available for patients who are sensitive to iron, such as iron drops for babies and vitamin supplements for children (check for added dyes and flavoring). Of course, these sources of iron may need to be taken more often for adults to benefit.

B Vitamins Taking B vitamins before conception can help prepare the body for pregnancy. B vitamins are extremely important throughout pregnancy and during lactation. For example, folic acid helps to prevent birth defects. B vitamins also help the body utilize key nutrients and work best when taken together, as in a B-complex supplement or a multivitamin, such as a prenatal supplement.

If B vitamins are irritating, they can be consumed alternatively in liver, grass-fed beef, whole and unrefined grains, brown rice, green leafy vegetables, nuts, beans, milk, eggs, fortified foods, and cereals (if tolerated). *See Chapter Two for more information on B vitamins.*

> *One study found that children of mothers who had a diet high in vitamin D during pregnancy had less asthma and allergies. The mothers also benefited from vitamin D, as well as Omega 3 fatty acids.*

Stress and Pregnancy

The IC/BPS patient is used to controlling the stress in her life in order to keep symptoms quiet. Pregnancy is the time to take even more control, because stress causes the release of certain chemicals in the body. These chemicals can affect both a baby's physical and emotional health. Extra stress can be avoided by living with a regular schedule and sleeping pattern, as well as practicing stress reduction exercises. Babies seem to adjust to people and situations better when their mother keeps to a regular schedule during pregnancy.

The effects of stress and the different types of stress that may occur during pregnancy have been studied. For example, one study on the effects of music on a fetus showed soft music is very good for a baby while loud music is not. When loud music was aimed at a mother's abdomen, the fetus actually urinated. Another study demonstrated a common stress: working pregnant women are often placed under additional work demands as they prepare to take their maternity leave. Reading current research and information on pregnancy can provide valuable information and guidelines.

Exercise and Good Body Mechanics

Pregnancy is a time to try to stay strong and flexible. Some IC/BPS patients feel better than usual and are, therefore, more motivated to exercise. However, pregnancy is not the time for patients to take on new forms of challenging exercise. IC/BPS patients may be susceptible to muscle and/or bladder pain from too many repetitions of an exercise, holding a position for too long, over stretching muscles, and/or performing jarring movements. Trying to keep up with other pregnant women who do not have IC/BPS should not be a goal. Comfort and avoidance of fatigue should be a goal.

Following recommended gentle exercise to increase flexibility and strengthen the neck and lower back muscles can help patients carry their babies during and after pregnancy. Strength and flexibility in these areas are especially important in late-stage pregnancy when the extra weight, the relaxation of smooth muscle, and shift in the pelvis change the body's balance. Changes in the lower body affect the legs and feet, and leave the upper body with less support (most IC/BPS patients already have some compromise in their lower bodies due to the muscle weakness in their pelvic regions). Women in general may experience fatigue, fluid retention, leg cramps and pressure, including pressure on the pelvic floor. Cramping in the feet and legs can often be relieved with regular flexion, extension and rotation exercises of the feet. Calcium supplements (which have become controversial) and/or calcium-rich foods can also help to control cramping in the legs and feet. Walking and/or swimming can improve circulation.

Always talk to a doctor before beginning any new exercise regime and be aware of exercises and movements that should be avoided as pregnancy progresses. Don't wait until the last trimester to begin an exercise regime. A patient with low back problems before pregnancy should inform her doctors, because she may become vulnerable to cystitis, especially when her body's balance changes. Low-back strengthening is often prescribed. Strengthening in general and following the suggestions in *Chapter Three* can be helpful. Be sure to consult your doctor first.

Kegel Exercise

Women are sometimes advised to prepare their pelvic floor for delivery with Kegel exercises. Kegel exercises are intended to help women strengthen and improve voluntary control over their pelvic muscles. Most IC/BPS patients cannot contract their pelvic floor muscles or start and stop their urine stream without pain. Voiding can bring relief and the interruption of stopping can interfere. Kegel exercises are also related to orgasm. Doctors and therapists may promote the benefits of Kegel to their patients both sexually and preventively, but performing pelvic floor exercises is often not possible without triggering pelvic floor pain.

Pelvic floor exercises to strengthen the supporting muscles of the bladder and urethra are also prescribed to control incontinence that sometimes occurs with pregnancy. Pelvic floor strengthening may, or may not, work for incontinence during pregnancy, but incontinence usually goes away after delivery. If the IC/BPS patient decides to try Kegel exercises, she should keep her abdominal muscles relaxed when tightening her pelvic floor muscles. She should also avoid holding her breath. If Kegel exercises are agreeable, they should begin before the last trimester, but they should be discontinued immediately if they cause bladder and pelvic floor pain. Again, most IC/BPS patients cannot and should not tolerate or try Kegel exercises.

Massage and Muscle Therapy during Pregnancy

Some IC/BPS patients just feel better all over with the hormones during pregnancy. However, many pregnant women can benefit from massage and muscle therapy. Gentle "bodywork" or massage can help to prevent tension, discourage muscles from shortening, encourage circulation, and reduce fluid retention, all of which may add to muscle and bladder pain in patients. Of course, it is important to discuss any type of hands-on therapy with a doctor before pursuing this option.

During the last trimester some women with IC/BPS and other chronic conditions experience an increase in muscle pain and even the best therapies may not be as helpful as before. Following the general advice for pain relief, such as wearing support hose, using good ergonomics (supporting both the upper and lower back while sitting), and avoiding shoes or sandals with a negative heel can help to distribute body weight more evenly and provide better support.

Urinary Tract Infections

Hormonal changes during pregnancy cause the muscle tone of the urinary system to relax. At the same time, hormonal changes cause the kidneys to produce more urine. These physical changes in bladder function make a woman more vulnerable to bladder infections. Experts suggest that the IC/BPS patient have a urinalysis each prenatal visit. There are two factors that can contribute to an undetected urinary tract infection. First, the patient may have difficulty distinguishing IC/BPS symptoms from those of a bladder infection, and second, the pregnant woman doesn't always feel the symptoms of an infection. If there's ever any question of infection, it's vital to contact the doctor. Infected urine can affect the baby.

Naturally, no one wants to take antibiotics during pregnancy, and for many IC/BPS patients, antibiotics can mean bladder pain, frequency, yeast infections, and other allergic reactions. If you are prone to bladder infections, it may be advisable to establish a plan and discuss antibiotic treatment with your doctor in the beginning of pregnancy. This can help to avoid explanation and perhaps conflict later if there is an infection. (Macrobid is sometimes the antibiotic of choice during pregnancy.)

As a woman becomes larger with pregnancy, she sits with her buttocks and pelvis rolled back and under in a posterior position due to the extra weight carried in the front of her body. Some doctors have suggested that catching a urine specimen in this position can cause urine to run back into the vagina and, therefore, contaminate the catch. Using an alternative position while voiding may help a woman to get a cleaner catch and void more completely. To find an alternative position while sitting, sit as far back on the toilet seat as possible, lifting your buttocks up in the back, and opening your legs out so you can lean forward. This seated posture brings the upper body forward over the pelvis, allowing abdominal muscles to rest and the bladder to empty more fully and more directly into the specimen bottle. If a urine catch tests positive for infection, ask to give another specimen to double check. The doctor can also confirm infection with a catheter specimen.

Yeast Infections

The normal acid environment of the vagina changes as vaginal secretions increase during pregnancy. These changes plus the increase of hormones contribute to yeast infections. Using prevention with diet by reducing sweets and refined carbohydrates, as well as taking tolerated probiotics may help to reduce yeast in the large intestine where it can flourish with constipation. (Probiotics are also thought to be good for the baby's immune system.) Prevention also includes staying dry, wearing skirts and cotton underwear, and avoiding tight pants, leggings, and pantyhose.

A yeast infection during pregnancy can be treated with over-the-counter drugs, but it's necessary to notify your doctor and discuss treatment first. Yeast infections mostly occur late in pregnancy when constipation can intensify.

Constipation

To help prevent constipation during pregnancy, avoid refined grains and sugar, and eat plenty of fiber. Fiber is necessary to keep constipation in check, and fresh vegetables and fruit are good sources of fiber and contain important vitamins and minerals. However, grains work the best to encourage elimination. Whole wheat bread (watch out for added rye and vinegar) and cereals that contain the maximum amount of bran provide good fiber. Oat bran is another very good source and can be sprinkled on hot or cold cereals, added to cottage cheese, or cooked in various dishes. It's necessary to drink an adequate amount of water after eating a meal prepared with bran or other high fiber ingredients.

Another way to prevent constipation is to take a probiotic and a fiber drink daily. However, because fiber can interfere with vitamin absorption, it's necessary to take vitamin supplements at least one hour before taking a fiber supplement. Patients with constipation IBS, and/or PFD may not do well with fiber drinks and laxatives. (Only natural laxatives are advised during pregnancy.) Fiber will only add to the bulking that already exists in these patients, therefore, oils may be preferable to soften stools, or patients may find that probiotics work just fine. A small new study has shown that probiotics may also reduce the incidence of gestational diabetes which occurs in 8 out of 100 pregnant women.

Some patients find they can tolerate Klaire Labs "Pro-biotic Complex, 5+ Billion CFU's." This is one of the purest probiotics available and the contents of the capsule can be emptied into cool water if necessary.

Acid Reflux and Heartburn

Some experts suggest that eating a small amount of fatty food 30 minutes before a meal can help to reduce stomach acid and aid digestion. A doctor may recommend an over-the-counter medication. Tums is considered safe and may work best for the IC/BPS patient who experiences bladder pain with other acid-reduction medications. It is necessary to consult your doctor before taking over-the-counter medications.

Nausea

According to some experts women who get adequate vitamin B-6 and complex carbohydrates (whole, unrefined grains), and avoid a diet too high in protein may reduce nausea during pregnancy. However, B-6 supplements are usually a bladder irritant for IC/BPS patients, so patients may want to get their B-6 from foods such as whole grains, almonds, and fish. (Certain fish should be avoided while pregnant. All fish should be bought from a known source. Both canned Wild Planet Albacore and canned Vital Choice Salmon filter out mercury and heavy metals.)

Migraines

Hormones may cause migraine headaches during pregnancy. Hormonal sensitivity is very individual, but the IC/BPS patient who experiences hormone related migraines with her menstrual cycle may react to the same hormones during her pregnancy. However, the IC/BPS patient may instead experience relief without the "ups and downs" of her monthly cycle, or at least find improvement after the first trimester when progesterone levels even off and estrogen levels rise. Again, it is necessary to keep your doctor informed of problems, especially if you are accustomed to taking medications for your migraines.

With your doctor's permission, trigger point therapy or acupuncture may help to relieve migraine headaches.

Delivery and IC/BPS

IC/BPS patients don't usually experience a worsening of bladder symptoms during delivery, even though the bladder is affected during the different types of delivery. However, patients should plan and be prepared to deal with IC/BPS symptoms that could occur with, and/or after, delivery. Researching and networking with other patients are very important. *Refer to the* Interstitial Cystitis Survival Guide *by Robert M. Moldwin, M.D., for more information about delivery.*

Some patients choose to have a dula in the delivery room to act as an advocate for their special needs. A dula is a female who provides physical and emotional assistance to a woman and her family through pregnancy, delivery, and postpartum.

C-Section Delivery

When the IC/BPS patient has a C-section, there's anesthesia and other medications to consider. There are decisions to make about being catheterized, as well as bladder-care after surgery. Networking with other patients who have had a C-section delivery will help. Working closely with your doctor and hospital staff is also necessary. *See Surgeries and Hospital Stays, Chapter Five and refer to the "Pregnancy Diaries" for more information on C-Section and vaginal deliveries.*

Vaginal Delivery

There are different factors to consider with a vaginal delivery. Although the IC/BPS patient may not have to worry about the medications needed during a C-section, she must consider how she will deal with her bladder during labor, an episiotomy (an incision made to increase the size of the vagina), and how she will feel after delivery.

Patients often need to pace and empty their bladders frequently to reduce the pain and pressure of bladder symptoms. Although a catheter may help some patients during labor, it may be an irritant to others or a limitation to those who must move around. Other considerations with a vaginal delivery include the possibility of needing repeated pelvic exams, drugs to induce labor, and of course, pain medication.

IC/BPS Pain after Pregnancy

Pelvic floor pain and spasms may occur after delivery, but patients often enjoy the lasting effects of estrogen after childbirth. The benefits of estrogen can last anywhere from six weeks to a few months. Patients who breast feed may not experience IC/BPS symptoms, migraines, or FMS until they finish breast feeding their babies.

Patients who do not breast feed can get back on their medications. Although not considered a standard treatment, some doctors suggest that women with IC/BPS or migraine symptoms may be helped by using an estradiol patch or topical gel until hormones are balanced. Other experts suggest that because progesterone levels are so high during pregnancy, mothers may be helped by taking natural progesterone to fight postpartum symptoms after they have delivered. Progesterone is not always tolerated by IC/BPS patients.

Some women have their first experience of IC/BPS symptoms after giving birth. Many different reasons have been speculated, such as hormonal changes and surgery when women have had a C-section. Because IC/BPS can be so unpredictable, patients should plan to have assistance with their babies until their symptoms are back in check.

Episiotomy

An antispasmodic, pain medication, an ice pack, and sometimes a catheter can be used to reduce inflammation, swelling, and pelvic floor spasms after an episiotomy. Warm baths are also helpful to soothe and aid the healing process. However, it's necessary to first ask the doctor if a bath is okay.

Caesarean Postpartum

As with other surgeries a patient must have time to recover. The IC/BPS patient may need IC/BPS treatments and extra help with her new lifestyle. She also may need to work closely with her doctor and/or a dietitian to get the needed nutrition to rebuild her body and take care of her new baby after surgery.

Breast Feeding

When breast feeding, women must continue with good nutritional habits. Breast feeding requires equal, if not more good nutrition than pregnancy. Although breast feeding is beneficial to a baby, new mothers with IC/BPS may need to get back on a diet for IC/BPS or take medication to control symptoms. Some mothers try to give their babies a little breast milk before switching to a bottle formula.

Breast feeding requires a woman to do with less sleep. Experts suggest that the new mother with IC/BPS express her milk so another person can feed the baby while mom gets some sleep.

Coping with a Newborn

It takes a lot of energy to cope with a newborn. The lack of sleep, occasional postpartum depression, the possibility of IC/ BPS symptoms returning, the lifting, holding, and bending, plus the partner and other children in need of your attention can make life difficult. Planning for all of these factors and how to take care of yourself will help.

A massage after delivery may help relieve the physical changes your body has endured with pregnancy and delivery. Rearranging the physical environment in your home to suit your needs will also help. Asking for help from family and friends, and taking enough time to get back to a normal pace is necessary. Comparing yourself to other new mothers without IC/BPS should be avoided.

If there is any doubt that you are not physically and/or emotionally recovering from childbirth, you should ask to be tested for anemia and hypothyroidism. Pain and fatigue should not be taken for granted. IC/BPS experts recommend that a patient not wait until her first postpartum appointment to deal with concerns.

Resources

Information and Consultation

Chronic Pain Research Alliance (CPRA)
(Formerly: The Overlapping Conditions Alliance)
www.endwomenspain.org

Harvard Women's Health Watch
www.health.harvard.edu/newletters
(800) 829-5921 • (904) 445-4662 (Canadian subscribers)

National Sjögren's Syndrome Association (NASSA)
www.sjogrenssyndrome.org • (800) 395-NSSA (6772)

Sjögren's Syndrome Foundation
www.sjogrens.org • (800) 475-6473

Vulvodynia Foundations
www.nva.org • (301) 299-0775

Randy Birken, M.D.
www.birkenmedicalaesthetics.com • (281) 419-3231

Products

Slippery Stuff
www.slipperystufflubes.com • (800)-759-7883

Books

Secret Suffering: How Women's Sexual and Pelvic Pain Affects Their Relationships, Susan Bilheimer and Robert J. Echinberg, M.D. www.instituteforwomeninpain.com.

Healing Painful Sex: A Woman's Guide to Confronting, Diagnosing, and Treating Sexual Pain, Debra Coady and Nancy Fish, M.S.W., M.P.H.

Ending Female Pain: A Woman's Manual, Isa Herrera, M.S.P.T. and C.S.C.S.

The Pregnant Couples' Guide to Working Together, Isa Herrera, M.S.P.T. and C.S.C.S.

The Book of Love, Laura Berman, Ph.D.

Please Understand: The Interstitial Cystitis Guide for Partners, Gaye and Andrew Sandler, Ph.D. and Molly Hanna Glidden and William Glidden (May be ordered from The IC Network)

Chapter Nine

LIVING WITH IC/BPS: A PARTNER'S PERSPECTIVE

Twenty-seven years ago, when I first began dating my wife, I did not know much about IC/BPS, a chronic disease that has changed both our lives. Like most people in the late 1980s, I had little awareness of IC/BPS. And, like most men, I had limited understanding of how problems can affect a woman's body.

The words "Interstitial Cystitis" (IC) were foreign to me when we first began to date. My future wife had lots of energy, kept up with me during long walks, and ate all of the same foods that I enjoyed. I did not even notice that she needed to use the bathroom an unusual amount of times.

Being a typical person, my future wife did not initially want me to know that she was not feeling well. As our relationship progressed, I realized that she did have to use the bathroom more frequently than most people and that she seemed to be in some kind of pain. As we grew more comfortable with each other, Gaye began to verbalize what she was physically experiencing. These problems related to gynecological and urological problems, which I knew nothing about, and she kept seeing doctors who never seemed to help.

We became engaged and my future wife finally saw the right doctor, a wonderful urologist in New Orleans, Kathleen Walsh, who made the correct interstitial cystitis diagnosis. I was at her side when the diagnosis was made. (This was long before the term "bladder pain syndrome" was used.) Although she received the diagnosis, it felt like it was also my diagnosis because of the implications that it had for our future lives together.

Shortly after we were married, I realized that, if I was going to keep my sanity for the rest of my life, I was going to have to adapt and make some changes. I continued to accompany my wife to doctor appointments and I vividly remember when a doctor told both of us that the disease would not necessarily get worse in the future. That knowledge made me feel much better. I also began to accept the fact that the IC/BPS was not going to go away, and that I was going to have to find ways to cope.

I have a Master's Degree in clinical psychology and have been employed as a therapist or in an administrative role in the health-care field for over 30 years. Some might say that my professional training would make it easier for me to cope with a wife who has IC/BPS. From an objective point of view, it is true that I know a great deal about clinical ways to help families deal with disease.

Yet, because this disease affects both of us, I have many sub-jective feelings that are hard to ignore. Giving advice to others is much easier than incorporating that advice into my own life. This makes me just like other family members of IC/BPS patients. Even after living with IC/BPS for years, I do not always handle my feelings in constructive ways. I get angry, feel sorry for myself, and feel sad.

At times I have felt resentful about vacations and special dinners that had to be canceled. Like many partners of IC/BPS patients, I have had to change my expectations about what life with my wife should be like. I have even perceived my wife as a bladder and forgotten she has other aspects to her identity.

Once we were married, I also became aware of my wife's other physical problems, described in earlier chapters in this book, which often accompany IC/BPS, such as chemical sensitivity and irritable bowel syndrome (IBS). In some ways, I have found these issues to be more troublesome to me than IC/BPS. Over time, my wife has incorporated lifestyle changes such as exercise and dietary modifications, and has found the right combination of bladder instillations so that her flare-ups are less frequent and intense. I know that my wife's IC/BPS will never completely go away but at some emotional level I feel that there is some control that we both have with this disease.

On the other hand, I can never predict when my wife will run into scents or chemicals once we leave our home. On several occasions, we have had to switch hotels late at night after a long day of travel because of perfumes and chemicals. Also, her dietary modifications for irritable bowel syndrome, such as a gluten-free diet, restrict our restaurant options even more than her IC/BPS. At times, I become extremely frustrated and angry when these inconveniences interfere with my plans and expectations.

IC/BPS is not just a physical disease. It has powerful emotional side effects, and it changes the way a family must live day-to-day. It can interfere with everything from one's sex life to a party invitation from the boss, to the weekly trip to the grocery store. But, because most IC/BPS sufferers look healthy and are often young, it is difficult for significant others to accept the seriousness of the condition.

After dealing personally with all of these issues for many years, I have learned many ways to make life with an IC/BPS patient not only manageable, but also satisfying and rewarding in all the ways we want our marriages and families to be satisfying and rewarding. This is what I would like to tell other partners and family members coping with IC/BPS. But families need help and support because this disease will require great sacrifice and change. Partners can run away or get trapped in denial, or they can go too far in the other direction and get so involved in taking care of their IC/BPS partners, they forget their own needs—even their own identities. Caregivers often need care as much as the patients.

There are some helpful coping tips I will offer later in this chapter. But first, before I plunge in with advice, I want to look at the coping process more broadly, in a developmental and family context, so that the ways to live more reasonably with IC/BPS are considered in proper perspective.

What do I mean? Family members, just like the IC/BPS patient, will go through different stages of dealing with the disease, depending on their age, their situation, their awareness of what is actually happening with the patient, and of course the patient's particular needs.

Everything will change, and continue to change. Even if you or others in your family are coping well with IC/BPS, this may change as you enter new phases of your life or deal with stressful situations. The birth of a baby, the IC/BPS patient's inability to continue working, cancellation of an anticipated family vacation, or when children reach adolescence—these can spark new stress. But stressful times do not always involve major life changes. For example, when the IC/BPS patient starts following the recommended diet, the relationship will be pressured. You may have to give up favorite foods and restaurants.

Once family members learn to accept and expect change, they'll be able to cope and adapt better, no matter how much their lives are altered. I like to think of living with an IC/BPS patient as a marathon, not a sprint. IC/BPS, as a chronic illness, is something family members and the patient will have to deal with over time.

Look at the contrast of a chronic illness such as IC/BPS with an acute illness like the flu. When a child has the flu, for instance, family members must make changes in their lives—call the doctor, stay home from work, get prescriptions filled, make chicken soup. But in a few days the child is well, and everyone returns to their normal routine. With IC/BPS, family members will have to continually make adjustments, year-after-year.

Learning to Accept IC/BPS

Given the constantly changing dynamics of the family, the most important thing families of IC/BPS patients can do is accept the disease and accept that it will continue to change their lives over time. Acceptance can be complex, and it does not happen overnight. In many cases IC/BPS comes on gradually, and some patients can have symptoms for a long time before they are diagnosed and treated. Patients and family may have been dealing with heavy-duty stress long before the IC/BPS is diagnosed. You can expect the acceptance process to be quite different for the patient and the family members. The IC/BPS patient may feel relieved at finally getting a diagnosis for her or his symptoms and learning that treatment is available. At the same time, family members may feel more confusion than relief.

IC/BPS may differ from other chronic diseases that have no cure, but it also is similar. In dealing with such diseases, denial always comes before acceptance. Most every family member, I believe, should expect to experience some denial about the reality and implications of IC/BPS. It may be useful to view this denial as the first stage of acceptance.

I have learned many ways to ease the acceptance process along. The most helpful thing is learning as much as possible about IC/BPS. I recommend accompanying your partner to the urologist or urogynecologist. This accomplishes several things. By listening to the doctor, you can better understand what your partner is going through. You will get an opportunity to gain information about IC/BPS, ask questions, and help your spouse remember the doctor's instructions.

And, just by being present, you are supporting your partner. Sometimes doctors do not take the symptoms of IC/BPS patients seriously, so your presence is a powerful confirmation that your partner is indeed suffering. Although education has greatly improved, there are still far too many doctors and nurses who are uneducated about IC/BPS, so you, as a family member, will need to be an advocate for the patient. Patients can also get complacent. They may hesitate to seek treatment. Going with your partner helps her or him avoid passivity.

I also do get satisfaction when I can help my wife during an appointment by confirming her symptoms to skeptical doctors. But it's interesting how our perceptions of a doctor are sometimes different. There have been several instances in which I thought a doctor was great and my wife has had the opposite reaction. Once I tried to convince her to see a urogynecologist who lived near our home because of my concern when she has had to drive long distances after a bladder instillation. But she made it clear to me that she would rather go out of her way to see a supportive doctor who respects her opinions about IC/BPS. I think that I now finally understand the frustration and anger that has built up in her through the years in regards to insensitive doctors.

Learning as much as possible is crucial when dealing with IC/ BPS. In some strange way, there are patients and family members who would find it easier to deal with a more dangerous disease like cancer simply because it is better accepted and brings sympathetic and compassionate responses from others. Although awareness has vastly improved, IC/BPS is not well-known, and because men do not understand the way the symptoms present in the female body, it is easy to think that the patient should be able to control them. At some level, most of us fall into the trap of believing that people with urinary problems should be able to use willpower to control their symptoms.

There is nothing scarier than the unknown. With IC/BPS, the more you know, the easier things will be. Being present and eager to learn can also put you in touch with encouraging news. I remember feeling comforted when the doctor told us that IC/BPS does not have to get worse with age.

Taking Control

Families of IC/BPS patients can cope better by gaining as much control as possible over their environment. One major way to take control is to plan ahead. Make planning in advance a way of life in every possible situation. There are many ways to accomplish this.

- Find bathrooms in advance. We know where every public bathroom is located in the cities in which we have lived. We will often modify our route during routine car trips according to the location of bathrooms. While IC/BPS is not a psychosomatic disease, IC/BPS sufferers, like everyone else, are more likely to need to use the bathroom when they are anxious. Locating bathrooms eases anxiety on many levels.
- Learn to be flexible and give up strict time schedules. With practice, you can learn to allot more time than you will probably need for every activity. Always have a back-up plan ready.

- We have lived in large cities and always try to avoid highway rush hour traffic. Sitting in a traffic jam without access to a bathroom is our worst case scenario. We even try to schedule flights on weekends because there is less traffic on the way to the airport.
- We always make other people aware of the problems (i.e., need for frequent bathroom stops and dietary requirements) associated with IC/BPS prior to taking a road trip with them. We will not travel with those who are not accepting of this disease.
- Schedule trips or special events when there is a good chance that the IC/BPS patient will feel strong. Many women with IC/BPS have symptoms that get worse according to their menstrual cycle. Do not plan events when symptoms are most severe.
- When flying, it is often helpful to fly in the late afternoon or early evening so that the IC/BPS patient can have a good bladder-safe breakfast and lunch prior to the flight (the bladder is most active in the morning and early afternoon). It is always a good idea to bring food (if allowed) on the plane and sit in the aisle seat in order to avoid disturbing other passengers during frequent trips to the bathroom.
- Staying with other people during vacations can be problematic. Families and friends, however well-meaning, often do not understand the unique problems of the IC/BPS patient. Sharing a bathroom and food is not ideal. The patient can go hungry if the dinner prepared is not bladder-safe. Relationships can become strained when IC/BPS becomes an issue in another person's home. We often chose to stay in a hotel and rent a car. The privacy of a hotel room allows my wife to rest and pace herself during a trip. Having a car enables us to find a variety of restaurants or go to a grocery.
- A major way IC/BPS sufferers can take control of their own lives is by following the recommended diet, which my wife discusses in other chapters. The diet truly lessens symptoms for most patients. But it is restrictive, so a partner can be extremely supportive just by helping the patient stick with it. This was tough for me because I have been told that I do

not eat to live, I live to eat. I love to eat out, so I did not like ruling out restaurants that do not serve what my wife can eat. We no longer go to French restaurants or share a bottle of wine over dinner. But because I accept that the diet is important and that my wife needs my support, these sacrifices are easier to make. When my wife feels better, I feel better. Now I know everything about my wife's diet. I read labels carefully and look at restaurant menus on-line before trying a new restaurant. I will often cook my favorite meals for dinners so I feel psychologically like my food needs are being met. We work together as a team to help her stay on the diet. Working as a team will help both you and your partner feel more in control and avoid stress.

Dealing with Feelings

I have felt the gamut of emotions since my wife began suffering with IC/BPS. What is particularly confounding about the condition is that it stirs up so many conflicting feelings.

For example, I love my wife and want to help her feel healthy and feel good about herself, but no matter what I do, she is often still uncomfortable or in pain, and still has to go to the bathroom all the time. I feel as if everything I try to do is useless. So I feel helpless, then angry, then guilty for feeling angry. This cycle of feelings will be all-too-familiar to family members of IC/BPS patients. I think that it is important to reassure patients and family members that these emotions are natural and normal. A partner who feels such conflict is not a bad person.

The best way to deal with intense feelings is to acknowledge they exist and deal with them constructively. It does not help to try to cover them up or keep them inside until they come out in inappropriate ways, such as kicking a door. Good communications among family members is essential to this process.

Sometimes I also need to look at what is going on in my life when I become angry. Three years into our marriage I often became very angry with my wife because of the extra things I needed to do such as the major grocery shopping. As I think about this time in my life rationally, I realize that there were other dynamics going on. I had the boss from hell, hated my job, and had a long work commute. What was going on was not Gaye's IC/BPS, because I had already been living with this disease and nothing had changed. I needed to put things in perspective.

Overall, I have dealt with negative feelings by learning to be realistic, especially about my expectations. I do not build up high hopes about anything. Then, when things do work out, I am pleasantly surprised. I have learned to be more realistic by increasing my knowledge of IC/BPS and giving myself some time. I have adjusted my thinking and my expectations for our lives together. In the process, my anger has gone away.

Early on, it is so important to alter your expectations of your partnership and your life, together and separately. I used to envision us taking vacations together, enjoying delicious dinners out, and going to parties and special events. I have had to realize that my wife will not always feel well enough to be by my side. And, I have accepted the even harder reality that she may have to cancel plans at the last minute. Changing my expectations has helped me deal with my anger and frustration.

Let me point out that changing expectations does not guarantee that you will never feel angry again. I feel like I have come a long way in accepting my wife's IC/BPS, but I still get angry at her. When we have plans to go on a trip, I accept that it may have to be canceled, but I sometimes still get mad if it happens.

It's important to never compare persons with IC/BPS to other healthy persons. Not only is this unfair, it will increase frustrations. In many cases, it is not realistic to expect persons with IC/BPS to work. It is also not realistic for a patient's partner to get his hopes up for sex on a certain night.

I am a firm believer that counseling can be valuable to families living with IC/BPS. Talking with a professional can give you an objective look at ways you can de-stress your life, take control of the things you can, and handle your negative feelings. My wife and I went to a social worker together and our lives are better as a result. We learned how to handle our negative feelings more effectively. For example, we made the joint decision to pay someone to do our laundry rather than getting upset over how and when it got done.

Family Dynamics

In my experience, dealing with IC/BPS caused my wife and me to take on distinct roles in the relationship. I began to see myself as the caregiver and my wife as the patient—or even worse, as a bladder. Of course, I am more than a caregiver, and my wife is more than a patient, even though we often assume those roles.

It is emotionally dangerous for family members of IC/BPS patients to define themselves in such rigid ways. I am more than a caregiver. I am a professional in the field of geriatrics. I am a friend to many people. I have outside interests other than IC/BPS. I have had to learn that I can still have a good day on a weekend when my wife is sick in bed. I can go out and enjoy myself without her. Luckily for me, my wife encourages me to do this.

It works the other way, too. Family members need to help the IC/BPS patient see her or his role as more than the "sick person" or victim. My wife has many interests, talents, and dimensions. She is a whole person.

Both the patient and partner must find ways to exercise their independence of the other at times and remember they are separate people with unique interests. This is something I continually work on in my life. It is easy for couples dealing with a chronic disease to become too intertwined in each other. This results in major problems. With an IC/BPS patient who has no children, the partner may fall even more easily into a caregiver role. Some partners are so immersed in caring for their partners that they do not take care of themselves and their own needs.

At the other extreme, some IC/BPS partners run away. When an IC/BPS patient gets divorced, I suspect that the disease was not the only problem. In many cases, the couple may have had communication problems and other difficulties that the condition brought to the surface.

Even when a couple has a solid relationship, they are constantly under stress because the partner of an IC/BPS patient must carry a heavier load in the marriage. And, IC/BPS also can cause financial problems if the patient can no longer work. The partner may have to take more responsibility for household management, errands, chores, and child-rearing. Good communication, making sure one's needs are met, and recognizing your identity as a person separate from the disease and caregiving role are essential in alleviating such stress.

In the extended family of an IC/BPS patient, expect to encounter misunderstanding and denial, even from mothers and mother-in-laws whom you might think would be compassionate. Even family members who accept the disease will do so at different stages. It can be helpful to bring these family members to a support group meeting.

Giving family members time also helps. After a while, people do understand. But family gatherings can be a challenge, especially on holidays and special occasions when the IC/BPS patient's absence, pain, or diet may become hot-button issues. Adjusting your own expectations and promoting constant education of all family members can help.

How families with children can best deal with IC/BPS depends on many factors: ages of the children, how long a parent has suffered with IC/BPS, and how well a family communicates and handles emotions. Working to maintain a good relationship is extremely important if a couple has children when IC/BPS is diagnosed. In these situations, the partner may feel overwhelmed with responsibility. Children need complete and total understanding, and a parent with IC/BPS will find supplying these qualities difficult at times.

Whatever the case in a particular family, children must always be told that their parent is sick so that they do not develop false expectations or misunderstanding. You cannot hide the illness anyway, because even small children will be aware that something is wrong. They need to know that there will be times when their mother, or father, needs peace and quiet and may not be available to them. Young children can be extremely helpful when a parent is experiencing symptoms. They seem to have a sympathetic understanding. However, the same child may react quite differently upon reaching adolescence.

Children do have higher expectations than adults. So when planning with children, it helps to concentrate on brief high-quality activities and outings that the IC/BPS patient can handle. Even with IC/BPS, you can still be a good mother or father and make your children feel loved and secure.

Improving Communication

As I think about ways to cope with the presence of IC/BPS in a family and keep stress down and a marriage strong, I continually come back to the importance of good communication. Keeping communication open and effective is a basic strategy helpful in solving every problem that comes up when dealing with IC/BPS.

We are not mind readers and good relationships are possible only when both parties tell each other what their needs are and feel that these needs are being met. They cannot do this without good communication, which can be a challenge even under the best of circumstances.

I sometimes think that I am the perfect husband because of the trials and tribulations that I have to put up with because of IC/BPS. But my wife sometimes tells me that I am being "dutiful" when I shop and help out. This response usually makes me feel unappreciated. It also serves as a cue to me that something is wrong and that I need to have further conversation with her. In most instances, she will finally verbalize that I was not listening and understanding her feelings.

I need to continually remind myself to ask my wife how she is feeling and then I need to take the time to really listen to what she is saying. This is not an easy task because I have lived with over 20 years of flare-ups and am so used to them that I guess I take them for granted. Unfortunately, each flare-up is painful and is not something that she is able to minimize or ignore. I do not always take the time to stop what I am doing and ask her how she is feeling and what she needs at the time, and this can make my wife feel like I do not care. Of course, communication is a two-way street and the patient also shares the responsibility of verbalizing feelings to her or his partner.

Good communication needs to be top-priority within a marriage, and outside of it, too. Everyone has to have someone other than their spouse to talk with. This is usually more difficult for men than for women. I speak from experience. Discussing my wife's illness is not what I want to do with other men while drinking a beer and watching a ball game. Fortunately, I happen to work with nurses, who are very supportive and helpful to me.

My wife learned early in her illness how vital it is for IC/BPS patients to find a good support group. I define a "good" support group as one which emphasizes positive coping and mutual help rather than pity. It helps to encourage your partner to find such a support group, and go with her occasionally. Talking with other people in the same situation can be invaluable.

Dealing with Other People

One of the many challenges of living with IC/BPS is coping with the reactions of other people. I cannot say this enough: IC/BPS is not easily understood. How do you explain needing time off from work to go to a doctor's appointment? How do you respond when new friends invite you and your partner to a dinner party?

I feel it is best to tell friends and family members the truth about IC/BPS. Being truthful does not mean telling everyone everything or expecting them to completely understand. You can decide in advance how much is appropriate to reveal in certain situations. I have told my employers that my wife has a chronic bladder disease, and I often receive supportive, positive responses. My perception is that people are much more understanding of the IC/BPS diet now than when Gaye was diagnosed in the 1980s, because of the increased publicity of other dietary restrictions such as gluten, peanuts, salt, etc.

It has also helped my wife and me to stay on the same social program. We keep our expectations of our social life toned down and decide together what we are going to do. Even so, going to parties and the homes of friends is hard. If we accept an invitation, we have to somehow tell the hosts that my wife has a chronic disease and can only eat certain foods. This can be tough. I remind myself that friends who do not understand are not really good friends.

Partner Support

Over the years, I've had the opportunity to speak with many IC/BPS patients and their significant others at conferences and support groups. Many of these patients have verbalized that they have supportive partners who love them. I've also heard stories from the viewpoint of their partners. These individuals seemed to be very happy and well adjusted, despite the challenges of living with IC/BPS.

Becoming a supportive partner does not mean becoming consumed with IC/BPS. Each person in a healthy relationship needs to find ways to meet their own needs and desires. The challenge is finding the best balance in terms of time and emotional commitment when one member of this relationship has IC/BPS. I believe that it is possible for the partner to feel fulfilled while doing and saying the things that a patient also needs. I hope that reading this chapter assists you in reaching that goal.

REFERENCES

Journals/Magazines/Newspapers

A short circuit in your nervous system, *Fibrmomyalgia Network,* January 2010

Are myofascial trigger points contributing to your pain?, *AFSA Update,* November 2009

Autotomic dysfunction in FMS, *Fibromyalgia Network,* January, 2002

Beauty secrets, *The Green Guide,* Spring 2008

Better results with acupuncture, *Remedies,* March 2010

Building blocks, consider these eco-friendly options when you build or remodel, *Natural Home,* July/August 2007

Can you smell that smell?, *Chicago Tribune,* January 8, 2008

Conference Report: American Urological Association 2008, *The IC Optimist,* Summer 2008

Cracking the code, Picking the best plastics for storing your food and drink, *Green Guide,* Spring 2008

Endometriosis and IC: The evil twins, *ICA Update,* Summer 2008

Getting the best hormonal mix, *Whole Living,* June 2010

Get to know Neem, *Remedies,* December 2010

Ethics from farm to table, *Foods and PLU Codes,* September 9, 2010

Facial pain, headaches and pelvic discomfort, *Fibromyalgia Network,* April 2009

Fire in the belly: Whole health report, *Whole Living,* June, 2010

50 simple health tips, *Body & Soul,* November 2009

50 ways to eat sustainably, *Whole Living,* August 2010

Gluten intolerance, *Chicago Tribune,* September 6, 2009

Got Allergies? Try these alternative foods for good health, *Chicago Tribune,* June 3, 2009

Green dry cleaning, *Good Housekeeping,* January 2011

Global cooling, *Whole Living,* July/August 2010

Guided imagery for Women with Interstitial Cystitis: Results of a prospective, randomized controlled pilot study, *The Journal of Alternative and Complementary Medicine,* Volume 14, 2008

Head and neck pain caused by myofscial trigger points, *Fibromyalgia Network,* April 2007

How sex hormones, aging and sleep influence fibro, *Fibromylgia Network,* January 2010

IC Guidelines, *ICA Update,* Summer, 2010

ICA takes IC message to International Pelvic Pain Society Meeting, *ICA Update,* Nov/Dec 2004

IC: Expert Opinions, *Interstitial Cystitis Association,* Volume 1

Identifying and treating sources of fatigue, *Fibromyalgia Network,* July 2004

Is IC really on your nerves?, *ICA Update,* Spring 2011

It's complicated but this gynecologist is untangling all the pelvic pain knots, *ICA Update,* 2012

Join us for a progressive holiday dinner, *ICA Update,* Fall 2009

Jump over treatment hurdles, *ICA Update,* Spring 2010

Medications and supplements, *Dr. Andrew Weil's guide to heart health*

Myofascial pain syndrome, *Fibromyalgia Network,* January 2007

Nanotechnology: the next small thing?, *Delicious Living,* March 2010

New approaches, new devices for pelvic floor therapy, *ICA Update,* Spring 2008

Nontoxic pest control, *The Green Guide,* July/August 2005

Pelvic pain and Trigger points, *Fibromyalgia Network,* October, 2007

Physical therapy for IC goes mainstream with more techniques, more education, *ICA Update,* Spring 2005

NIDDK meeting ignites new research focus, *ICA Update,* Fall, 2008

Possible gene or genes for IC/PBS/CPPS, *Children's Hospital Boston,* Issue 1, January 2008

Preventing baby's allergies, *Parents,* June 2012

Probiotics' potential for IC, *ICA Update,* Summer 2011

Providers put focus on multidisciplinary pelvic pain practice, *ICA Update,* Winter 2010

PVC shower curtains, *The Green Guide,* Winter 2009

Power of probiotics, *Better Nutrition,* January, 2009

Real men do get IC. And when they do, it's a rough ride, *ICA Update,* Fall, 2010

Recent developments in BPS/IC, *Urology News,* July/August 2008

Rekindle your sexuality, *ICA Update,* Winter 2009

Shine on healthy glow, *Remedies,* 2010

Sleep, pain, dopamine and grey matter loss, *Fibromyalgia Network,* October 2007

Some things old, plenty new, some things borrowed, ICA Update, Winter 2010

Stay nourished, fit and comfortable, *ICA Update,* Winter, 2011

Stress and your looks, *Real Simple,* November 2013

Tame your bladder, *ICA Update,* Winter 2009

Tea for good health, *Delicious Living,* October, 2009

The ICA Treatments and Medications Guide, *Interstitial Cystitis Association*

The latest on gluten-free living, *Better Nutrition,* January, 2009

The role of diet and IC, *ICN Special Report On Diet,* Summer 2004

The right and wrong way to treat pain, *Time,* February 28, 2005

This is your body on exercise, *Better Homes And Garden,*August, 2012

Tiffany's cupboard, *Green Guide,* Fall 2008

Time to grow, Put the green back into gardening, *Green Guide,* Summer 2008

Thwarting mast cells to stop inflammation, *ICA Update,* Fall 2008

Time to exercise, *Better Home And Gardens,* March, 2008

Treating you as an individual and the rationale for multidrug therapy, *Fibromyalgia Network,* January 2009

Treatment choices for pregnancy and childbirth, *ICA Update,* Winter 2011

Two groundbreaking IC research studies published, *ICA Update,* April/May 2004

What exercise can do for you, *A Special Health Report From Harvard Medical School*

What popular meds can be doing to you, *Fibromyalgia Network*, April 2011

What to expect from physical therapy, *ICA Update*, April/May 2005

What's new in neurostimulation?, *ICA Update*, Spring 2008

Why it hurts more for FM Patients, *Fibromyalgia Network*, July 2010

Why overdoing it causes symptom flares, *Fibromyalgia Network*, October 2010

XMRV accelerates scientific interest in CFS, *The CFIDS Association of America*

You've come a long way, IC treatment, *ICA Update,* Summer, 2010

Books

Brookoff, D., 2008, *Genitourinary pain syndromes: Interstitial cystitis, chronic prostatitis, pelvic floor dysfunction and related disorders*

Laumann, B., 1998, *A taste of the good life,* Freeman Family Trust Publications, Tustin, CA

Sant, G., 1997, *Interstitial cystitis,* Lippincott-Raven, Philadelphia, PA

Schapiro, M., 2007, *Exposed, the toxic chemistry of everyday products and what's at stake for American power,* Chelsea Green Publishing, White River Junction, Vermont

Websites

Clinical phenotyping in chronic prostatitis/chronic pelvic pain syndrome and interstitial cystitis: A management strategy for urologic chronic pelvic pain syndromes, www.medscape.com

How can we manage multifactorial pain?, www.medscape.com

IBS study, *Ohio State University News Release*, August 2010

IC and pudendal neuralgia, nerve inflammation and pelvic pain, *ICA Website*, August 2011

Mystery of migraines, www.healthiernashville.com

No safe haven, www.emagazine.com

Pain and pH: Acid-sensing channels (ACIS) may play a role in bladder pain syndrome (BPS), *Uro Today*, February 2012

Pregnancy and interstitial cystitis, painful bladder syndrome, *Uro Today*, February 2007

INDEX

ABOUT THE AUTHORS

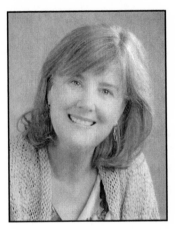 GAYE GRISSOM SANDLER is an author and educator living in Nashville. Gaye holds a B.A. in Humanities from New College of California and completed one of the first alternative programs for holistic educators at Holistic Life University in San Francisco. After training with movement pioneer, Judith Aston, and becoming a practitioner of muscle and movement re-education, she worked for many years in physical therapy and wellness clinics. While living in Boston, Gaye and her husband, Andrew, facilitated an IC support group at the Newton-Wellesley Hospital and, in conjunction with the ICA, produced an exercise video for IC patients. They have also given separate workshops and presentations at ICA National Meetings and had a column on the IC Network, called *LifeStyles*. In 2000, Gaye and Andrew published *Patient to Patient: Managing Interstitial Cystitis and Overlapping Conditions*. Other publications include *Stretch into a Better Shape: Stretching and Strengthening for Interstitial Cystitis and Fibromyalgia Patients*, which was co-authored with physical therapist, Merrilee Kullman, and *The Interstitial Cystitis Guide for Partners*, which Gaye and Andrew co-authored with former IC support group leader Molly Hanna Glidden and her husband William Glidden.

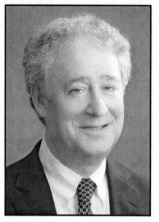

ANDREW SANDLER is the Executive Director of Park Manor and Chief Executive Officer of Abe's Garden, a national model of residential living and day care programs for those affected by Alzheimer's and dementia. Andrew holds three graduate degrees, including a Masters of Health Administration from Tulane University, a Ph.D. in Special Education from the University of New Orleans, and a Masters of Arts in Clinical Psychology from Farleigh Dickinson University in Teaneck, New Jersey. He received his undergraduate degree in Psychology from DePauw University in Greencastle, Indiana. He has written numerous journal articles that have appeared in publications such as *Advances in Special Education*, the *Journal of Behavioral Education*, *The Urban Review*, and the *American Journal of Occupational Therapy*. His article *American Tragedy: New Orleans Under Water* was published in *Callaloo* in 2007. Andrew has served as a board member of the Gulf States Association of Homes and Services for the Aging and as the President of the Alzheimer's Association New Orleans Regional Advisory Committee.

ABOUT THE ARTISTS

Ellen Hermanos Braunstein is originally from New York City and makes her home outside of Boston. Both a clinical social worker and an artist, she splits her time working with patients and painting abstractions motivated by mood and balance. Ellen's art has shown in galleries in New York, Boston, and New Orleans, and has been featured in home decorating magazines and on various television and movie settings. She and Gaye met at an IC support group 26 years ago and have been best friends ever since. Ellen's IC went into remission after discovering the benefits of a gluten-free diet.

Katherine Rutledge grew up in New Orleans and made Baton Rouge her home after receiving a B.A. in Fine Arts at Louisiana State University. Katherine continued her studies in painting in both New Orleans and Baton Rouge. Her art presently hangs in museums and private collections, institutes, and various galleries in Louisiana, and she was recognized in the *Marquis Who's Who in American Women in 2004*. After damage to her bladder during a hysterectomy, she had to have two surgeries months apart. During that time she experienced how all-encompassing to her mind and bladder the pain was. Fortunately, the surgeries were successful. Katherine and Gaye were best friends in high school and have continued their friendship to this day.